Assessment

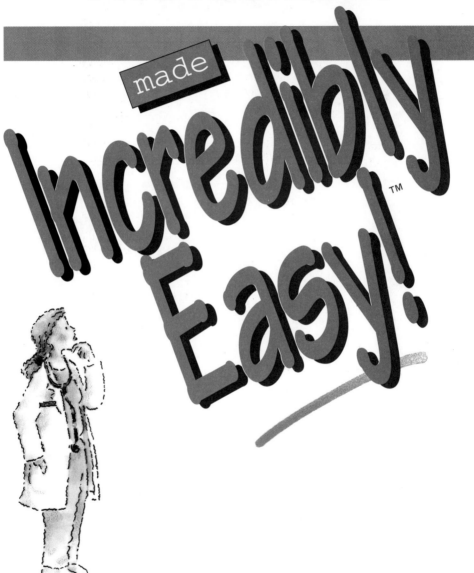

made Incredibly Easy!™

Springhouse Corporation
Springhouse, Pennsylvania

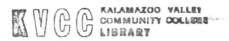

MAY 1 4 1998

Staff

Executive Director
Matthew Cahill

Editorial Director
Patricia Dwyer Schull, RN, MSN

Art Director
John Hubbard

Clinical Manager
Judith A. Schilling McCann, RN, MSN

Senior Editor
Michael Shaw

Clinical Editors
Ann M. Barrow, RN, MSN, CCRN (project manager); Clare M. Brabson, RN, BSN; Pamela A. Kovach, RN, BSN; Karen E. Michael, RN, MSN; Marybeth Morrell, RN, CCRN, Carla Roy, RN, BSN

Editors
Marylou Webster Ambrose; A. T. McPhee, RN, BSN; Dianna P. Sinovic; Patricia Wittig

Copy Editors
Cynthia C. Breuninger (manager), Karen C. Comerford, Brenna H. Mayer

Designers
Matie Patterson (project manager), Lorraine Lostracco (book designer), Joseph Clark

Photographer
John Gallagher

Illustrators
Barbara Cousins, John Cymerman, Jackie Facciolo, Jean Gardner, Linda Gist, Frank Grobelny, Bob Jackson, Cynthia Mason, John Murphy, Robert Neumann, Judy Newhouse, Bot Roda, Mary Stangl

Typography
Diane Paluba (manager), Joyce Rossi Biletz, Phyllis Marron, Valerie Rosenberger

Manufacturing
Deborah Meiris (director), T.A. Landis, Otto Mezei

Production Coordinator
Margaret A. Rastiello

Editorial Assistants
Carol Caputo, Beverly Lane, Mary Madden

Indexer
Barbara Hodgson

Photo credits
Custom Medical Stock Photo
 Basal cell carcinoma, malignant melanoma, squamous cell carcinoma, p. 59; *scabies, vitiligo,* p. 60; *contact dermatitis, psoriasis, urticaria,* p. 61; *herpes, impetigo,* p. 62
Photo Researchers, Inc.
 Eczema, p. 61
Phototake
 Lupus erythematosus, p. 60
Carroll H. Weiss
 Kaposi's sarcoma, p. 59; *telangiectasia,* p. 60; *candidiasis, tinea corporis,* p. 62

The clinical treatments described and recommended in this publication are based on research and consultation with nursing, medical, and legal authorities. To the best of our knowledge, these procedures reflect currently accepted practice. Nevertheless, they can't be considered absolute and universal recommendations. For individual applications, all recommendations must be considered in light of the patient's clinical condition and, before administration of new or infrequently used drugs, in light of the latest package-insert information. The authors and the publisher disclaim any responsibility for any adverse effects resulting from the suggested procedures, from any undetected errors, or from the reader's misunderstanding of the text.

Printed in the United States of America.

IEASSESS-021097

℞ A member of the Reed Elsevier plc group

Library of Congress Cataloging-in-Publication Data

Assessment made incredibly easy.
    p. cm.
  Includes index.
  1. Nursing assessment — Handbooks, manuals, etc. I. Springhouse Corporation.
  [DNLM: 1. Nursing Assessment — handbooks.
  2. Physical Examination — nurses' instruction.
  WY 49 A846 1997]
RT48.A876 1997
616.07'54— dc21
DNLM/DLC   97-7655
ISBN 0-87434-888-9 (alk. paper)   CIP

Direct gift 4-29-98 $29.95

Contents

Contributors and consultants

Betty Rosemary Akers, RN, MSN, FNP
Assistant Professor of Nursing
State University of West Georgia
Carrollton

Joan Brogan, RN, MN
Director of Nursing and Health Education
North Idaho College
Coeur d'Alene

Renée Cantwell, RN, MSN, CPHQ
Clinical Quality Management Specialist
Department of Veterans Affairs
Medical Center
Philadelphia

Mary J. Christian, RN,C, MSN
Clinical Educator
The Graduate Hospital
Philadelphia

Paula Cleanthous, RN, MN
Nursing Instructor
North Idaho College
Coeur d'Alene

Ellie Z. Franges, RN, MSN, CNRN, CCRN
Director
Neuroscience Services
Sacred Heart Hospital
Allentown, Pa.

Nancy Haynes, RN, MN, CCRN, TNCC
Assistant Professor of Nursing
Saint Luke's College
Kansas City, Mo.

Nancy M. Holloway, RN, MSN
Critical Care Consultant
Nancy Holloway and Associates
Orinda, Calif.

LuAnn Joy, RN, BA, CCRN
Clinical Education and Management
Consultant
Staff Nurse
Postanesthesia Care Unit
Lutheran Medical Center
Wheat Ridge, Colo.

Mary Dirr Kostenbauder, RN, CNM, MEd, MSN
Instructor
Seminole Community College
Sanford, Fla.

Nancy L. Kranzley, RN, MS
Pulmonary Clinical Nurse Specialist
The Christ Hospital
Cincinnati

Virginia Lee, RN, MSN, MBA
Assistant Professor
Nursing Program
Northern Virginia Community College
Annandale

Kay L. Luft, RN, MN, CCRN, TNCC
Assistant Professor of Nursing
Saint Luke's College
Kansas City, Mo.

Denise Netz, RN, CRNP, MSN, ANP
Nurse Practitioner
Dublin (Pa.) Medical Center

Mary S. O'Neill, RN, MSN
Assistant Professor
State University of West Georgia
Carrollton

Beverly A. Reno, RN,C, MSN
Associate Professor
Northern Kentucky University
Highland Heights

Carla Roy, RN, BSN
Staff Nurse
Medical Intensive Care Unit
The Graduate Hospital
Philadelphia

Linda Roy, RN, CRNP, MSN, CCRN
Faculty, School of Nursing
Nurse Practitioner, Cardiology
Allegheny University Hospital
Philadelphia

Jan Schlaier, RN, MS, CS, FNP
Assistant Professor of Nursing
University of Tampa (Fla.)

Barbara A. Strande, RNCPN, MA, MSN
Assistant Professor
Western Kentucky University
Bowling Green

Kimberly Zalewski, RN, MSN
Staff Nurse
St. Luke's Hospital
Bethlehem, Pa.

Bonnie Zauderer, RN, MS, CNS
Assistant Professor of Clinical Nursing
University of Texas
Houston Health Science Center
School of Nursing

Foreword

Nurses are becoming increasingly responsible for obtaining health histories and performing physical examinations in clinics, hospitals, and patient's homes. They simply never know when they'll need to perform a particular assessment skill, one they might seldom — or *never* — have used in the past.

For instance, I was asked on the spur of the moment one day to teach a physical assessment workshop to nurse practitioners. Now, I ordinarily would have felt completely confident in my assessment skills. On this particular occasion, however, I was asked to teach how to perform an extensive neurologic assessment, including tests of all the cranial nerves. I had been working in an outpatient clinic with young, healthy people and only rarely needed to perform an extensive neurologic examination.

How I wish *Assessment Made Incredibly Easy* — with its clear and easy-to-read language, plentiful photographs, abundant illustrations, and concise summaries of key points — had been around then! I could have easily reviewed important details about the neurologic examination and been ready for any question the students threw my way.

The book might have arrived too late for me to use in that workshop, but it's just in time for you. *Assessment Made Incredibly Easy* can help you master the difficult and sometimes intimidating art of history-taking and physical assessment.

Every topic — from examining the retina to percussing liver borders to auscultating for a pericardial friction rub — is described step by precise step.

Assessment Made Incredibly Easy is divided into chapters based on body systems. Each chapter begins with a review of anatomy and physiology. Next, it covers common complaints and lists questions to ask when obtaining a health history. From there, it describes the assessment skills needed for the specific body system as well as common abnormal findings.

Assessment Made Incredibly Easy's key feature is its user-friendly format. Each chapter begins with a summary of major concepts. Checklists on just about every page make it easy to spot the most important points. Memory joggers (the fancy term is mnemonics) help you understand and remember difficult points. And the informal writing style makes learning fun.

Special logos throughout each chapter identify key information for practitioners and make it easy to find specific topics. For instance:

 Peak technique shows how to perform specific assessment techniques — perfect for when you need to prepare quickly for an unfamiliar examination.

 Advice from the experts offers pointers on refining history-taking and physical assessment skills such as differentiating a flat percussion note from a dull one.

 What does it all mean provides surefire guidelines for interpreting assessment findings quickly and easily; for example, how to determine possible causes of abdominal pain.

Finely detailed photographs and illustrations make it easy to understand difficult techniques and concepts. You'll find two full-color sections — one on identifying common skin disorders, the other on understanding and identifying heart sounds.

Mastering the art of physical assessment can be a challenging task. *Assessment Made Incredibly Easy* is a powerful and highly efficient tool that can help you become an assessment expert. Soon, you'll be percussing the liver, measuring diaphragmatic excursion, and performing neurologic examinations with ease and confidence.

I just know this book will be a welcomed, comforting companion on the job, and a resource you'll never want to be without.

Mary D. Knudtson, RN, MSN, FNP, PNP, CS
Assistant Clinical Professor
Director, Family Nurse Practitioner Program
College of Medicine
University of California, Irvine

Part I

Beginning the assessment

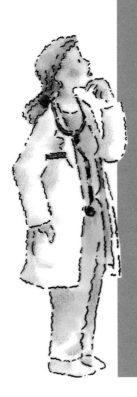

Health history

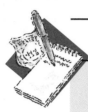

Just the facts

This chapter covers the first step in the patient assessment process: taking a health history. In this chapter, you'll learn:

♦ why a health history is performed

♦ how to communicate effectively with your patient while taking a health history

♦ what steps — from obtaining biographic data to reviewing body systems — make up a complete health history

♦ what questions to ask each step of the way.

Obtaining a health history

Knowing how to carry out an accurate assessment — from taking the health history through performing the physical examination — will help you uncover significant problems and plan your care appropriately. Assessment involves collecting two kinds of data: objective and subjective.

Objective data is obtained through observation and is verifiable. For instance, you may see a red, swollen arm in a patient who's complaining of arm pain. That observation can then be verified by someone else. Subjective data is provided by the patient and is based on what he says. For example, he might say, "My head hurts" or "I have trouble sleeping at night."

Exploring past and present

A health history is used to gather subjective data about the patient and to explore past and present problems. First, ask the patient about his general physical and emotional health, and then ask him questions about specific body systems and structures.

The accuracy and completeness of your patient's answers depend largely on your skill as an interviewer. Before you start asking questions, review the communication guidelines in the following sections.

Interviewing the patient

Before asking your first question, you'll need to set the stage, explain what you'll cover during the interview, and establish rapport with the patient. Here's how.

Settling in

- Choose a quiet, private, well-lit interview setting away from distractions. This will make it easier for you and your patient to interact and help the patient feel more at ease.
- Make sure that the patient is comfortable. Sit facing him, about 3′ to 4′ (0.9 to 1.2 m) away.
- Introduce yourself and explain that the purpose of the health history and assessment is to identify the patient's problem and provide information for planning his care.
- Reassure the patient that everything he says will be kept confidential.
- Tell the patient how long the interview will last, and ask him what he expects from the interview.

Watch what you say

- Assess the patient to see if language barriers exist. (See *Overcoming interviewing obstacles.*) For instance, does he speak and understand English? Can he hear you?
- Speak slowly and clearly, using easy-to-understand language. Avoid medical terms and clichés.
- Address the patient by formal name, such as Mr. Jones or Ms. Carter. Don't call him by his first name unless he asks you to. Treating the patient with respect encourages him to trust you and provides more accurate and complete information.

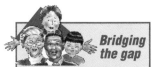

Bridging the gap

Overcoming interviewing obstacles

With a little creativity, you can overcome barriers to interviewing. For example, if a patient doesn't speak English, your facility may have a bank of interpreters you can call on for help. You might also find an interpreter among the patient's family members or friends. Just be sure to tell the interpreter to translate the patient's speech verbatim and not to change the meaning in any way.

Breaking the sound barrier

Is your patient hard of hearing? You can overcome this barrier, too. First, make sure the light is bright enough for him to see your lips move. Then face him and speak slowly and clearly. If necessary, have the patient use an assistive device, such as a hearing aid or an amplifier. If the patient uses sign language, see if your institution has a sign-language interpreter.

Look out for body language

- Listen attentively and make eye contact frequently. (See *Overcoming cultural barriers.*)
- Use reassuring gestures, such as nodding your head, to encourage the patient to keep talking.
- Watch for nonverbal cues that indicate the patient is uncomfortable or unsure about how to answer a question. For example, he might lower his voice or glance around uneasily.
- Be aware of your own nonverbal cues that might cause the patient to "clam up" or become defensive. For example, if you cross your arms, you might appear "closed off" from him. If you stand while he is sitting, you might appear superior. If you glance at your watch, you might appear bored or rushed, which could keep the patient from answering questions completely.

Know what I'm saying?

Observe the patient closely to see if he understands each question. If he doesn't appear to, repeat the question using different words or familiar examples. For instance, instead of asking, "Did you have respiratory difficulty after exercising?" ask "Did you have to sit down after walking around the block?"

Open up those questions

You might also use a different type of question. An open-ended question such as "How did you fall?" lets the patient respond more freely. (See *Two ways to ask.*) His response can provide answers to many other questions.

For instance, from the patient's answer, you might learn that he has fallen before, that he was unsteady on his feet, and that he fell before dinner. Armed with this information, you might deduce that he had a syncopal episode caused by hypoglycemia.

You can also ask closed questions. However, they require only a yes-or-no answer and generally don't provide extra information.

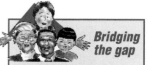

Bridging the gap

Overcoming cultural barriers

To maintain a good relationship with your patient, remember that his cultural behaviors and beliefs may differ from your own. For example, most people in the United States make eye contact when talking with others. However, people in a number of other cultures — including Native Americans, Asians, and Arabs — may find eye contact disrespectful or aggressive.

Communication strategies

Besides the tips listed above, seven special communication techniques — silence, facilitation, confirmation, reflection, clarification, summary, and conclusion — can help you make the most of your patient interview.

Two ways to ask

You can ask your patient two types of questions: open-ended and closed.

Open-ended questions

These questions require the patient to tell a kind of story about himself, expressing feelings, opinions, and ideas. They also help you gather more information than can be gathered with closed questions. Open-ended questions encourage a good nurse-patient rapport because they show you're interested in what the patient has to say. Examples of such questions include:
- Why did you come to the hospital tonight?
- How would you describe the problems you're having with your breathing?
- What lung problems, if any, do other members of your family have?

Closed questions

Closed questions elicit yes-or-no answers or one- to two-word responses. They limit the development of nurse-patient rapport. Examples of closed questions include:
- You came to the hospital tonight because of your breathing, right?
- Do you ever get short of breath?
- Are you the only one in your family with lung problems?

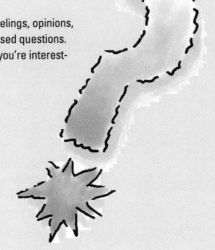

Silence is golden

Moments of silence during the interview encourage the patient to continue talking and give you a chance to assess his ability to organize thoughts. You may find this technique difficult; many people are uncomfortable with silence. The more you use it, however, the more comfortable with it you'll become.

Lead him on

Facilitation encourages the patient to continue with his story. Using such phrases as "please continue," "go on," or even "uh-huh" shows him that you're interested in what he's saying.

OK, now, to confirm...

Confirmation ensures that both you and the patient are on the same track. You might say, "If I understand you correctly, you said...," and then repeat the information the patient gave. This technique helps to clear up misconceptions you or the patient might have.

Check and reflect

Reflection — repeating something that the patient has just said — can help you obtain more specific information. For example, a patient with a stomachache might say, "I know I have an ulcer." You might repeat, "You know you have an ulcer?" And the patient might then say, "Yes. I had one before, and the pain is the same."

Clear things up

Clarification is used to clear up confusing, vague, or misunderstood information. For example, if your patient says, "I can't stand this," your response might be, "What can't you stand?" or "What do you mean by 'I can't stand this?' " This gives the patient an opportunity to explain his statement.

Sum it up

Summarizing is restating the information the patient gave you. It ensures that the data you've collected is accurate and complete. Summarizing also signals that the interview is about to end.

Bring it to a close

Conclusion allows the patient himself to end the interview. To accomplish this, use a statement like, "I think I have all the information I need now. Is there anything you'd like to add?"

Specific questions to ask

You've learned how to ask questions. Now it's time to learn the right questions to ask. A complete health history requires information from each of the following categories, obtained in this order:
1. biographic data
2. chief complaint
3. medical history
4. family history
5. psychosocial history
6. activities of daily living.

Biographic data

Start the health history by obtaining biographic information from the patient. Do this first; otherwise, you may forget once you become involved in details of the patient's health. Ask the patient for his name, address, telephone number, birth date, age, marital status, religion, and nationality. Find out who he lives with and the name and telephone number of a person to contact in case of an emergency.

Also ask the patient about his health care, including the name of his primary doctor and how he gets to the doctor's office. Ask if he has ever been treated for his present problem before.

Take the hint

Your patient's answers to basic questions can provide important clues about his personality, medical problems, and reliability. If he can't furnish accurate information, ask him for the name of a friend or relative who can. Be sure to document who gave you the information.

Chief complaint

The patient's chief complaint — for example, dizziness, rash, or dyspnea — is what causes him to seek health care. Document this information in the patient's exact words to avoid misinterpretation. Ask how and when the symptoms developed, what led the patient to seek medical attention, and how the problem has affected his life and ability to function.

To make sure you don't omit pertinent data, use the PQRST mnemonic device, which provides a systematic approach to obtaining information. (See *Exploring the chief complaint*, page 8.)

Medical history

Ask the patient about past or current medical problems, such as hypertension, diabetes, or back pain. Typical questions include:
• Have you ever been hospitalized? If so, when and for what reason?
• What childhood illnesses did you have?
• Are you under treatment for any problem? If so, what is the problem and who is your doctor?
• Have you ever had surgery? If so, when and for what reason?
• Are you allergic to anything in the environment or to any drugs? If so, what kind of allergic reaction do you have?
• Are you taking medications, including over-the-counter drugs such as aspirin, vitamins, and cough syrup? If so, how much do you take and how often do you take it? Do

Exploring the chief complaint

Use the PQRST mnemonic device to fully explore your patient's chief complaint. When you ask the questions below, you'll encourage him to describe his symptoms in greater detail.

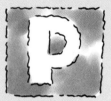  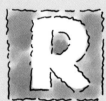 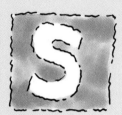 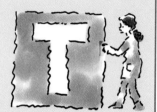

Provocative or palliative	**Quality or quantity**	**Region or radiation**	**Severity**	**Timing**
Ask the patient: • What provokes or relieves the symptom? • Does anything trigger the symptom; for example, stress, anger, or certain physical positions? • What makes the symptom worsen or subside?	Ask the patient: • What does the symptom feel like, look like, or sound like? • Are you having the symptom right now? If so, is it more or less severe than usual? • To what degree does the symptom affect your normal activities?	Ask the patient: • Where in the body does the symptom occur? • Does the symptom appear in other regions? If so, where?	Ask the patient: • How severe is the symptom? How would you rate it on a scale of 1 to 10, with 10 being the most severe? • Does the symptom seem to be diminishing, intensifying, or staying about the same?	Ask the patient: • When did the symptom begin? • Was the onset sudden or gradual? • How often does the symptom occur? • How long does the symptom last?

you use home remedies, such as homemade ointments or creams?

Family history

Questioning the patient about his family's health is a good way to uncover his risk of having certain illnesses. Typical questions include:
• Are your mother, father, and siblings living? If not, how old were they when they died? What was the cause of death?
• If they're alive, do they have diabetes, high blood pressure, heart disease, asthma, cancer, sickle cell anemia, hemophilia, cataracts, glaucoma, or other illnesses?

Psychosocial history

Find out how the patient feels about himself, his place in society, and his relationships with others. Ask about his occupation, education, financial status, and responsibilities. Typical questions include:
• How have you coped with medical or emotional crises in the past? (See *Asking about abuse*.)
• Has your life changed recently? What changes in your personality or behavior have you noticed?
• How adequate is the emotional support you receive from family and friends?
• Do you feel you have a responsibility to promote your own health? If so, how do you do this?
• How often do you exercise? How often do you eat a healthful diet?
• How close do you live to health care facilities, and can you get to them easily?
• Do you have health insurance?
• Are you on a fixed income with no extra money for health care?

Activities of daily living

Find out what is normal for the patient by asking him to describe his typical day. Be sure to include the following four areas in your assessment.

Diet and elimination

Ask the patient about his appetite, special diets, and food allergies. Can he afford to buy enough food? Who cooks and shops at his house? Ask about frequency of bowel movements and laxative use.

Exercise and sleep

Ask the patient if he has a special exercise program and, if so, why? Have him describe it. Ask how many hours he sleeps at night, what his sleep pattern is like, and whether he feels rested after sleep.

Work and leisure

Ask the patient what he does for a living and what he does during his leisure time. Does he have hobbies?

Use of tobacco, alcohol, and other drugs

Ask the patient if he smokes cigarettes. If so, how many does he smoke each day? Does he drink alcohol? If so,

---

Asking about abuse

Abuse can be emotional, sexual, or physical. Anyone can be a victim: a boyfriend or girlfriend, a husband or wife, an elderly parent, or a child. When taking a health history, be sure to ask two open-ended questions: When do you feel safe at home? When do you not feel safe?

Watch the reaction

Besides listening to the answer, watch how the patient reacts to the question. Is he defensive, hostile, confused, or frightened? Assess how he interacts with you and others. Does he seem withdrawn or frightened or show other inappropriate behavior? Keep his reactions in mind when you perform your physical assessment.

how much each day? Ask if he uses illicit drugs, such as marijuana or cocaine. If so, how often?

Patients may understate the amount they drink because of embarrassment. If you're having trouble getting what you believe are honest answers to such questions, you might try overestimating the amount. For example, you might say, "You told me you drink beer. Do you drink about a six-pack a day?" The patient's response might be, "No, I drink about half that."

Maintaining a professional outlook

Don't let your personal opinions interfere with this part of the assessment. Maintain a professional outlook, and don't offer advice. For example, don't suggest that the patient enter a drug rehabilitation program. That type of response puts him on the defensive and he might not answer subsequent questions honestly.

In addition, avoid saying things like, "The doctor knows what's best for you." Such statements make the patient feel inferior and break down communication. Finally, don't use leading questions such as "You don't do drugs, do you?" to get the answer you're hoping for. This type of question, based on your own value system, will make the patient feel guilty and might prevent him from responding honestly.

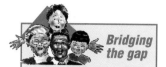

Bridging the gap

Overcoming communication problems in the elderly

An elderly patient may have sensory impairment, impaired memory, or a decreased attention span. If your patient is confused or has trouble communicating, you may need to rely on a family member for some or all of the health history.

Reviewing structures and systems

The last part of the health history is a systematic assessment of the patient's body structures and systems. Always start at the top of the head and work your way down the body. This helps keep you from skipping any areas. When questioning an elderly patient, remember that he may have difficulty hearing or communicating. (See *Overcoming communication problems in the elderly.*)

Asking the right questions

Information gained from a health history forms the basis for your care plan, enabling you to distinguish physical changes and devise a holistic approach to treatment. As with other nursing skills, you can improve your interviewing technique only with practice, practice, and more practice.

Here are some key questions to ask your patient about each body structure and system. (See *Evaluating a symptom*, page 12.)

Head first

Do you get headaches? If so, where are they located, and how painful are they? How often do they occur, and how long do they last? Does anything trigger them, and how do you relieve them? Have you ever had a head injury? Do you have lumps or bumps on your head?

Eye to eye

When was your last eye examination? Do you wear glasses? Do you have glaucoma, cataracts, or color blindness? Does light bother your eyes? Do you have excessive tearing, blurred vision, double vision, or dry, itchy, burning, inflamed, or swollen eyes?

An earful

Do you have loss of balance, ringing in your ears, deafness, or poor hearing? Have you ever had ear surgery? If so, why and when? Do you wear a hearing aid? Are you having pain, swelling, or discharge from your ears? If so, has this problem occurred before and how frequently?

By a nose

Have you ever had nasal surgery? If so, why and when? Have you ever had sinusitis or nosebleeds? Do you currently have nasal problems causing breathing difficulties, frequent sneezing, or discharge?

Into the mouth and down the throat

Do you have mouth sores, a dry mouth, loss of taste, a toothache, or bleeding gums? Do you wear dentures, and do they fit? Do you have a sore throat, fever, or chills? How often do you get a sore throat, and have you seen a doctor for this?

Do you have difficulty swallowing? If so, is the problem with solids or liquids? Is it a constant problem or does it accompany sore throat or another problem? What, if anything, makes it go away?

Evaluating a symptom

Your patient is vague in describing his chief complaint. Using your interviewing skills, you discover his problem is related to abdominal distension. Now what? This flowchart will help you decide what to do next, using abdominal distension as the patient's chief complaint.

Question the patient to identify the symptom bothering him. Although he's vague about his chief complaint, he tells you, "My stomach gets bloated."

Form a first impression. Does the patient's condition alert you to an emergency? For example, does he say the bloating developed suddenly? Does he mention other symptoms occurring with it; for example, sweating or light-headedness — both signs of hypovolemia?

YES

NO

Take a brief history to gather more clues. For example, ask the patient if he has severe abdominal pain or difficulty breathing or if he ever had an abdominal injury.

Now, take a thorough history to get an overview of the patient's condition. Ask him about associated signs or symptoms. Note especially GI disorders that can lead to abdominal distension.

Perform a focused physical examination to quickly determine the severity of the patient's condition. Check for bruising, lacerations, changes in bowel sounds, or rigidity of the abdomen.

Now, thoroughly examine the patient to evaluate the chief sign or symptom and to detect additional signs or symptoms. Observe the recumbent patient for abdominal asymmetry. Inspect the skin, auscultate for bowel sounds, percuss and palpate the abdomen, and measure his abdominal girth.

Evaluate your findings. Are emergency signs or symptoms present, such as abdominal rigidity or abnormal bowel sounds?

YES

NO

Based on your findings, intervene appropriately to stabilize the patient. Notify the doctor immediately, place the patient in a supine position, administer oxygen, and start an I.V. line. GI or NG tube insertion may be necessary, as well as emergency surgery.

Review your findings to consider possible causes, such as cancer, bladder distension, cirrhosis, congestive heart failure, or gastric dilation.

After the patient is stabilized, review your findings to consider possible causes, such as trauma, large-bowel obstruction, mesenteric artery occlusion, or peritonitis.

Evaluate your findings and devise an appropriate plan of care. Position the patient comfortably, administer analgesics, and prepare the patient for diagnostic tests.

Up to your neck

Do you have swelling, soreness, lack of movement, stiffness, or pain in your neck? If so, did something specific cause it to happen such as too much exercise? How long have you had this symptom? Does anything relieve it or aggravate it?

Breath by breath

Do you have shortness of breath on exertion or while lying in bed? How many pillows do you use at night? Do you have pain or wheezing when breathing? Do you have a productive cough? If so, do you cough up blood-tinged sputum? Do you have night sweats?

Have you ever been treated for pneumonia, asthma, emphysema, or frequent respiratory infections? Have you ever had a chest X-ray or a tuberculin skin test? If so, when, and what were the results?

The heart of the matter

Do you have chest pain, palpitations, irregular heartbeat, fast heartbeat, shortness of breath, or a persistent cough? Have you ever had an electrocardiogram? If so, when?

Do you have high blood pressure, peripheral vascular disease, swelling of the ankles and hands, varicose veins, cold extremities, or intermittent pain in your legs?

Breasts in women ... and men

Ask women these questions: Do you perform breast self-examinations on a monthly basis? Have you noticed a lump, a change in breast contour, breast pain, or discharge from your nipples? Have you ever had breast cancer? If not, has anyone else in your family had it? Have you ever had a mammogram? When, and what were the results?

Ask men: Do you have pain in your breast tissue? Have you noticed lumps or a change in contour?

That queasy-stomach feeling

Have you had nausea, vomiting, loss of appetite, heartburn, stomach or abdominal pain, frequent belching, or passing of gas? Have you lost or gained weight recently? How often do you have a bowel movement, and what is the color, odor, and consistency of your stools? Have you noticed a change in your regular pattern? Do you use laxatives frequently?

Have you had hemorrhoids, rectal bleeding, hernias, gallbladder disease, or a liver disease such as hepatitis?

Going with the flow

Do you have urinary problems, such as burning during urination, incontinence, urgency, retention, reduced urinary flow, or dribbling? Do you get up during the night to urinate? If so, how many times? What color is your urine? Have you ever noticed blood in it? Have you been treated for kidney stones?

Reproduction review

Ask women: How old were you when you started menstruating? How often do you get periods, are they regular, and how long do they last? Do you have clots or pain? If you're postmenopausal, at what age did you stop menstruating? If you're in the transitional stage, what menopausal symptoms are you experiencing? Have you ever been pregnant? If so, how many times? What was the method of delivery? How many pregnancies resulted in live births? How many resulted in a miscarriage? Have you had an abortion?

What is your method of birth control? Are you currently involved in a long-term, monogamous relationship? Have you had frequent vaginal infections or a sexually transmitted disease? When was your last gynecologic examination and Pap test? What were the results?

Ask men: Do you perform monthly testicular self-examinations? Have you ever had a prostate examination and, if so, when? Have you noticed penile pain, discharge, or lesions or testicular lumps? What form of birth control do you use? Have you had a vasectomy? Are you currently involved in a long-term, monogamous relationship? Have you ever had a sexually transmitted disease?

Bones and muscles

Do you have difficulty walking, sitting, or standing? Are you steady on your feet, or do you lose your balance easily? Do you have arthritis, gout, a back injury, muscle weakness, or paralysis?

Brain function

Have you ever had, or do you now have, seizures? Do you ever experience tremors, twitching, numbness, tingling, or loss of sensation in a part of the body? (See *Tips for as-*

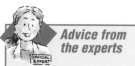
Advice from the experts

Tips for assessing severely ill patients

When the patient's condition doesn't allow a full assessment — for instance, if he is in severe pain — get as much information as possible from other sources. With severely ill patients, keep these key points in mind:

☑ Identify yourself to the patient and his family.

☑ Stay calm to gain their confidence and allay anxiety.

☑ Stay on the lookout for important information. For example, if a patient seeks help for a ringing in his ears, don't overlook his casual mention of a periodic "racing heartbeat."

☑ Avoid quick conclusions. Don't assume the patient's current complaint is related to his admitting diagnosis. Use a systematic approach and collect the appropriate information; then draw your own conclusions.

sessing severely ill patients.) Are you less able to get around than you think you should be?

Endocrine glands

Have you been unusually tired lately? Do you feel hungry or thirsty more than usual? Have you lost weight for unexplained reasons? How well can you tolerate heat or cold? Have you noticed changes in your hair texture or color? Have you been losing hair? Do you take hormone medications?

Blood

Have you ever been diagnosed with anemia or blood abnormalities? Do you bruise easily or become fatigued quickly? Have you ever had a blood transfusion?

Don't neglect emotional status

Do you ever have mood swings, anxiety, depression, inability to concentrate, or memory loss? Are you feeling unusually stressed? Do you ever feel unable to cope?

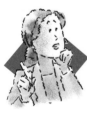

Quick quiz

1. Leading questions may initiate untrue or inaccurate responses because such questions:
    A. encourage short or vague answers.
    B. require an educational level the patient may not possess.
    C. prompt the patient to try to give the answer you're looking for.

Answer: C. Because of how they're phrased, leading questions may prompt the patient to give the answer he thinks you want to hear.

2. When obtaining a health history from a patient, ask first about:
    A. biographic data.
    B. chief complaint.
    C. health insurance coverage.

Answer: A. Take care of the biographic data first; otherwise, you might get involved in the patient history and forget to ask basic questions.

3. Silence is a communication technique used during an interview to:

    A. show respect.
    B. change the topic.
    C. encourage the patient to continue talking.

Answer: C. Silence allows the patient to collect his thoughts and continue to answer your questions.

4. Data is considered subjective if you obtain it from:

    A. what the patient says.
    B. your observations of the patient's actions.
    C. the patient's records.

Answer: A. Data from the patient's own words is subjective data. Objective data is based on your observations.

5. "If I understand you correctly, you said...," is an example of the interviewing technique:

    A. clarification.
    B. confirmation.
    C. reflection.

Answer: B. The phrase is an example of confirmation, a technique that can help clear up misconceptions you or the patient might have.

Scoring

☆☆☆ If you answered all five items correctly, bravo! You're our intrepid interviewer!

☆☆ If you answered three or four correctly, that's cool! You're our hip historian!

☆ If you answered fewer than three correctly, that's okay! This is only the first chapter. We've got lots more questions for you!

2

Fundamental physical assessment techniques

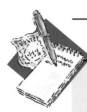

Just the facts

This chapter lays the groundwork for performing a physical assessment. In this chapter you'll learn:

♦ what equipment you'll need for the assessment and how to use it

♦ what to look for in your initial observation of the patient

♦ how to prepare your patient for the examination

♦ how to perform inspection, palpation, percussion, and auscultation.

A look at physical assessment

Once you've taken the patient's health history, proceed to the hands-on part of the assessment. During the physical assessment, you'll use your sense of sight, hearing, touch, and smell, along with a systematic approach, to collect information and complete the patient's health picture.

As you proceed through the physical examination, you can also teach your patient about his body. For instance, you can explain how to do a testicular self-examination or why the patient should monitor the appearance of a mole.

Think critically about what you find during the assessment and how it fits in with the patient's history. This evaluation will guide your plan of care.

Collecting the equipment

Before starting a physical assessment, assemble the equipment you'll need, including a stethoscope, a penlight, an ophthalmoscope, an otoscope, a percussion hammer, cotton balls, safety pins, and gloves. (See *Assessment tools.*)

Two heads are better than one

Use a stethoscope with a diaphragm and a bell. The diaphragm has a flat, thin, plastic surface that picks up high-pitched sounds such as breath sounds. The bell has a smaller, open end that picks up low-pitched sounds such as the heart sounds S_3 and S_4.

Other tools of the trade

You'll need a penlight to illuminate the inside of the patient's nose and mouth, cast tangential light on lesions, and evaluate pupillary reactions. An ophthalmoscope enables you to examine the internal structures of the eye, and an otoscope is used to look at the external auditory canal and tympanic membrane.

Other equipment includes a percussion hammer to evaluate deep tendon reflexes, cotton balls and safety pins to test sensation and pain differentiation, and gloves to protect the patient and yourself.

Performing a general survey

After assembling your equipment, move on to the first part of the physical assessment: forming your initial impressions of the patient and obtaining his baseline data, including height, weight, and vital signs. This information will direct the rest of your assessment.

Observing the patient

Many subtle clues to your patient's health can be found in his behavior and appearance. Carefully observe him for unusual behavior or signs of illness. Use this mnemonic checklist — *Some teams* — to help you remember what to look for:

Assessment tools

Tools used for assessment include:
• scale with height measurement
• stethoscope with two heads
• blood pressure cuff
• thermometer
• penlight
• ophthalmoscope and otoscope
• near-vision and visual acuity charts
• tuning fork
• nasal speculum
• percussion hammer
• clear metric ruler
• wooden tongue depressor
• safety pins and cotton balls
• gloves
• vaginal speculum
• cloth or paper tape measure
• skin calipers.

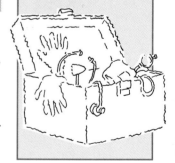

- **S**ymmetry — Are his face and body symmetrical?
- **O**ld — Does he look his age?
- **M**entation — Is he alert, confused, agitated, or inattentive?
- **E**xpression — Does he appear ill, in pain, or anxious?
- **T**runk — Is his body type lean, stocky, obese, or barrel-chested?
- **E**xtremities — Are his finger clubbed? Does he have joint abnormalities or edema?
- **A**ppearance — Is he clean and appropriately dressed?
- **M**ovement — Are his posture, gait, and coordination normal? Does he ambulate normally?
- **S**peech — Is his speech relaxed, clear, strong, understandable, and appropriate? Does it sound stressed?

Preparing the patient

If possible, introduce yourself to the patient before the assessment, preferably when he's dressed. Meeting him under less-threatening circumstances will decrease his anxiety when you actually perform the assessment.

Keep in mind that the patient may be worried you'll find a problem. He may also consider the assessment an invasion of his privacy because you're observing and touching sensitive, private, and perhaps painful body areas.

No surprises

Before you start, briefly explain what you're planning to do, why you're doing it, how long it will take, what position changes it will require, and what equipment you'll use. (See *Tips for assessment success.*) As you perform the assessment, explain each step in detail. A well-prepared patient won't be surprised or feel unexpected discomfort, so he'll trust you more and cooperate better.

Put your patient at ease, but know where to draw the line. Avoid inappropriate familiarity or touching during the examination. Humor can help put the patient at ease, but avoid sarcasm and keep jokes in good taste.

Get it down on paper

Document your findings up to now in a short, concise paragraph. Include only essential information that communicates your overall impression of the patient. For example, if your patient has a lesion, simply note it now. You'll describe the lesion in detail when you complete the physical assessment.

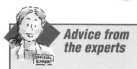
Advice from the experts

Tips for assessment success

Before starting the physical assessment, review this checklist.

☑ Eliminate as many distractions and disruptions as possible.

☑ Ask your patient to void before beginning the physical assessment.

☑ Wash your hands before and after the assessment — preferably in the patient's presence.

☑ Have all necessary equipment on hand and in working order.

☑ Make sure the examination room is well-lit and warm.

☑ Warm your hands and equipment before touching the patient.

☑ Be aware of your nonverbal communication and possible negative reactions from the patient.

Recording vital signs and statistics

Measurements of your patient's height, weight, and vital signs provide critical information about the patient's body functions. You'll need to be as accurate as possible with those measurements.

The first time you assess a patient, record his baseline vital signs and statistics. (See *Tips for interpreting vital signs*.) Afterward, take measurements at regular intervals, depending on the patient's condition and your facility's policy. A series of readings usually provides more valuable information than a single set.

Weight and height

Weight and height are important parameters for evaluating nutritional status, calculating medication dosages, and assessing fluid loss or gain. (See *Measuring height and weight*.) Take the patient's baseline height and weight so you can gauge future weight changes or calculate medication dosages in an emergency. Keep this information handy so you can refer to it quickly, if necessary.

Body temperature

Body temperature is measured in degrees Fahrenheit (F) or degrees Celsius (C). Normal body temperature ranges from 96.7° to 100.5° F (36° to 38° C), depending on the route used for measurement.

Hyperthermia describes an oral temperature above 106° F (41° C). Hypothermia describes a rectal temperature below 95° F (35° C).

From F to C and back again

To convert Celsius to Fahrenheit, multiply the Celsius temperature by 1.8 and add 32. (See *How temperature readings compare,* page 22.) To convert Fahrenheit to Celsius, subtract 32 from the Fahrenheit temperature and divide by 1.8.

Pulse

The patient's pulse reflects the amount of blood ejected with each heartbeat. To assess the pulse, palpate one of the patient's arterial pulse points and note the rate, rhythm, and amplitude (strength of the pulse). A normal pulse for an adult is between 60 and 100 beats per minute.

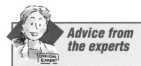

Advice from the experts

Tips for interpreting vital signs

Always analyze vital signs together because two or more abnormal values provide important clues to your patient's problem. For example, a rapid, thready pulse along with low blood pressure may signal shock.

Accuracy

If you obtain an abnormal value, take the vital sign again to make sure it's accurate. Remember that normal readings vary with the patient's age. For example, temperature decreases with age, and respiratory rate may increase with age or with an underlying disease process.

Individuality

Also remember that an abnormal value for one patient may be a normal value for another. Each patient has his own baseline values, which makes recording vital signs during the initial assessment so important.

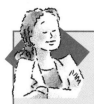

Peak technique

Measuring height and weight

Have the patient remove his shoes and dress in a hospital gown. Then use these techniques to measure his height and weight.

Balance the scale
Slide both weight bars on the scale to zero, as shown. The balancing arrow should stop in the center of the open box. If the scale has wheels, be sure to lock them before the patient gets on.

Measuring height
Ask the patient to turn his back to the scale. Move the height bar up over his head, and lift up the horizontal arm. Then lower the bar until the horizontal arm touches the top of his head. Now read the height measurement from the height bar.

Measuring weight
Slide the lower weight into the groove representing the largest increment below the patient's estimated weight. For example, if you think the patient weighs 145 lb (65.8 kg), slide the weight into the groove for 100 lb (45.4 kg).

Slide the upper weight across until the arrow on the right stops in the middle of the open box. If the arrow hits the bottom, slide the weight to a lower number. If the arrow hits the top, slide the weight to a higher number.

The patient's weight is the sum of these numbers. For example, if the lower weight is on 150, and the upper weight is on 11.5, the patient weighs 161.5 lb (73.2 kg).

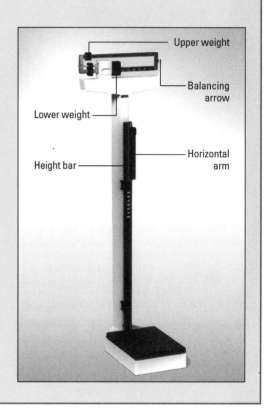

The radial pulse is the most easily accessible. (See *Pinpointing pulse sites*, page 23.) However, in cardiovascular emergencies, you may palpate for the femoral or carotid pulse. The vessels where you palpate for these pulses are larger and closer to the heart and more accurately reflect the heart's activity.

Feeling the beat

To palpate for a pulse, use the pads of your index and middle fingers. Press the area over the artery until you can feel pulsations. If the rhythm is regular, count the beats for 15 seconds and then multiply by 4 to get the number of beats per minute. If the rhythm is irregular or your patient has a pacemaker, count the beats for 60 seconds.

Keep in mind that to obtain an accurate rate, you should start at zero, not one. Starting the count at one adds

How temperature readings compare

You can take your patient's temperature four different ways. The chart below compares each route.

Route	Normal temperature	Reading time	Used for
Oral	97.7° to 99.5° F (36.5° to 37.5° C)	3 to 5 minutes	Adults and older children who are awake, alert, oriented, and cooperative
Axillary (armpit)	96.7° to 98.5° F (36° to 37° C)	11 minutes	Patients with impaired immune systems when infection is a concern; less accurate because it can vary with blood flow to skin
Rectal	98.7° to 100.5° F (37° to 38° C)	2 minutes	Infants, young children, and confused or unconscious patients; wear gloves and lubricate thermometer
Tympanic (ear)	98.2° to 100° F (36.8° to 37.8° C)	No set time; responds to subtle thermal changes and is unaffected by mouth breathing or patient movement	Adults and children, conscious and cooperative patients, and confused or unconscious patients; provides automatic timing through pushbutton device.

four extra beats when the pulse is counted for 15 seconds and multiplied by four.

Palpation pointers

Avoid using your thumb to count the pulse; the thumb has a strong pulse of its own. If you need to palpate the carotid arteries, avoid exerting a lot of pressure, which can stimulate the vagus nerve and cause reflex bradycardia. In addition, don't palpate for both carotid pulses at the same time. Putting pressure on both sides of the patient's neck can impair cerebral blood flow and function.

Off beat

When you note an irregular pulse, do the following:
• Evaluate whether the irregularity follows a pattern.
• Auscultate for the apical pulse while palpating for the radial pulse. You should feel the pulse every time you hear the heart beat.
• Measure the difference between the apical pulse rate and radial pulse rate, a measurement called the pulse

deficit. Measuring the pulse deficit allows you to indirectly evaluate the ability of each cardiac contraction to eject sufficient blood into the peripheral circulation.

From absent to bounding

You also need to assess the pulse amplitude. To do this, use a numerical scale or a descriptive term to rate or describe the strength. Numerical scales differ slightly between facilities, but the following scale is commonly used:
• *absent pulse:* not palpable, measured as 0
• *weak or thready pulse:* hard to feel, easily obliterated by slight finger pressure, measured as +1
• *normal pulse:* easily palpable, obliterated by strong finger pressure, measured as +2
• *bounding pulse:* readily palpable, forceful, not easily obliterated by pressure from the fingers, measured as +3.

Respirations

Along with counting respirations, be aware of the depth and rhythm of each breath. To determine the respiratory rate, count the number of respirations for 60 seconds. A rate of 16 to 20 breaths per minute is normal for an adult. *If the patient knows you're counting how often he breathes, he may subconsciously alter the rate. To avoid this, take his respirations while you take his pulse.*

Pay attention as well to the depth of the patient's respirations by watching his chest rise and fall. Is his breathing shallow, moderate, or deep? Observe the rhythm and symmetry of his chest wall as it expands during inspiration and relaxes during expiration. *Be aware that skeletal deformity, broken ribs, and collapsed lung tissue can cause unequal chest expansion.*

Accessory to the act ... of breathing

Use of accessory muscles can enhance lung expansion when oxygenation drops. Patients with chronic obstructive pulmonary disease or respiratory distress may use neck muscles, including the sternocleidomastoid, and abdominal muscles for breathing. Normal respirations are quiet and easy, so note any abnormal sounds, such as wheezing or stridor.

Blood pressure

Blood pressure measurements are helpful in evaluating cardiac output, fluid and circulatory status, and arterial re-

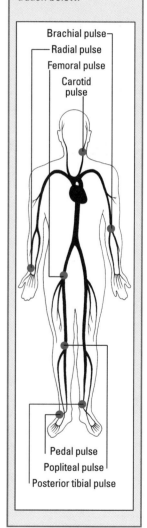

Pinpointing pulse sites

You can assess your patient's pulse rate at several sites, including those shown in the illustration below.

Brachial pulse
Radial pulse
Femoral pulse
Carotid pulse

Pedal pulse
Popliteal pulse
Posterior tibial pulse

sistance. Blood pressure measurements consist of systolic and diastolic readings. The systolic reading reflects the maximum pressure exerted on the arterial wall at the peak of left ventricular contraction. Normal systolic pressure ranges from 100 to 140 mm Hg.

The diastolic reading reflects the minimum systemic arterial pressure that occurs during left ventricular relaxation. This reading is often more significant than the systolic reading because it evaluates arterial pressure when the heart is at rest. Normal diastolic pressure ranges from 60 to 90 mm Hg.

Peak technique

Using a sphygmomanometer

Here's how to use a sphygmomanometer properly.
• For accuracy and consistency, position your patient with his upper arm at heart level and his palm turned up.
• Apply the cuff snugly, 1″ (2.5 cm) above the brachial pulse, as shown in the top photo.
• Position the manometer in line with your eye level.
• Palpate the brachial or radial pulse with your fingertips while inflating the cuff.
• Inflate the cuff to 30 mm Hg above the point where the pulse disappears.
• Place the bell of your stethoscope over the point where you felt the pulse as shown in the bottom photo. Using the bell will help you hear Korotkoff's sounds better.
• Release the valve slowly and note the point at which the Korotkoff 's sounds, indicating the pulse, reappear. The start of the pulse sound indicates the systolic pressure.
• The sounds will become muffled and then disappear. The last Korotkoff's sound you hear is the diastolic pressure.

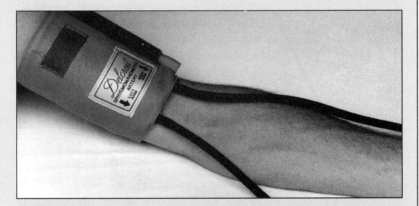

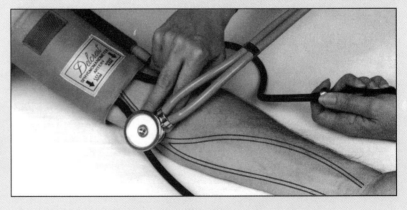

Unpronounceable but indispensable

The sphygmomanometer, a device used to measure blood pressure, consists of an inflatable cuff, a pressure manometer, and a bulb with a valve. (See *Using a sphygmomanometer*.) To record a blood pressure, the cuff is centered over an artery, inflated, and deflated.

As it deflates, listen with a stethoscope for Korotkoff's sounds, which indicate the systolic and diastolic pressures. (See *Tips for hearing Korotkoff's sounds*.) Blood pressure can be measured from most extremity pulse points. The brachial artery is used for most patients because of its accessibility.

Physical assessment techniques

During this part of the assessment, use drapes so that only the area being examined is exposed. Develop a pattern for your assessment, starting with the same body system and proceeding in the same sequence. Organize your steps to minimize the number of times the patient needs to change position. By using a systematic approach, you'll also be less likely to forget an area.

A tetrad of techniques

No matter where you start your physical assessment, you'll use four techniques, referred to as IPPA for *i*nspection, *p*alpation, *p*ercussion, and *a*uscultation.

The techniques are used in sequence except when performing an abdominal assessment. Because palpation and percussion can alter bowel sounds, the sequence for assessing the abdomen is: inspection, auscultation, percussion, and palpation. Let's look at each step in the sequence, one step at a time.

Inspection

Inspection uses vision, smell, and hearing to observe for normal conditions and deviations. It's also the most frequently used assessment technique. Performed correctly, inspection can often reveal more than other techniques.

Inspection is used when you first meet the patient and continues throughout the health history and physical examination aspects of your assessment. As you assess each

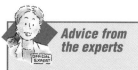

Advice from the experts

Tips for hearing Korotkoff's sounds

If you have trouble hearing Korotkoff's sounds, try to intensify them by increasing vascular pressure below the cuff. Here are two techniques you can use.

Raise the arm
Palpate for the brachial pulse and mark its location with a pen to avoid losing the pulse spot. Apply the cuff, and have the patient raise his arm above his head. Then inflate the cuff about 30 mm Hg above the patient's systolic pressure. Lower his arm until the cuff reaches heart level, deflate the cuff, and take a reading.

Make a fist
Position the patient's arm at heart level. Inflate the cuff to 30 mm Hg above the patient's systolic pressure, and ask him to make a fist. Have him rapidly open and close his hand about 10 times; then deflate the cuff and take the reading.

body system, observe for color, size, location, movement, texture, symmetry, odors, and sounds.

Palpation

Palpation requires you to touch the patient with different parts of your hand, using varying degrees of pressure. To do this, you need short fingernails and warm hands. Always palpate tender areas last. (See *Types of palpation*.) Tell your patient the purpose of your touch and what you're feeling with your hands.

Don't forget to wear gloves when palpating, especially when palpating mucous membranes or other areas where you might come into contact with body fluids.

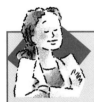

Peak technique

Types of palpation

The two types of palpation, light and deep, provide different types of assessment information.

Light palpation
Depress the skin ½" to ¾" (1.25 to 2 cm) with your finger pads, using the lightest touch possible. Perform light palpation to feel for surface abnormalities. Assess for texture, tenderness, temperature, moisture, elasticity, pulsations, superficial organs, and masses.

Deep palpation
Depress the skin 1½" to 2" (3.8 to 5 cm) with firm, deep pressure. If necessary, use one hand on top of the other to exert firmer pressure. Deep palpation is used to feel internal organs and masses for size, shape, tenderness, symmetry, and mobility.

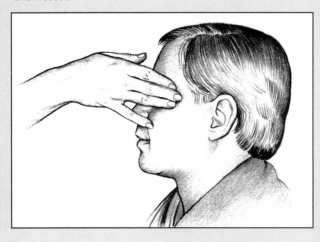

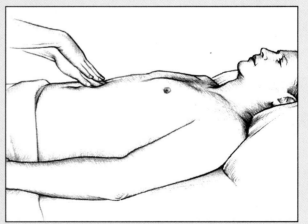

Check out these features

As you palpate each body system, evaluate the following features:
- texture: rough or smooth?
- temperature: warm, hot, or cold?
- moisture: dry, wet, or moist?
- motion: still or vibrating?
- consistency of structures: solid or fluid-filled?

Percussion

Percussion involves tapping your fingers or hands quickly and sharply against the patient's body, usually the chest or abdomen. (See *Types of percussion.*) The technique helps

Peak technique

Types of percussion

You can perform percussion using the direct or indirect method. Direct percussion elicits tenderness. Indirect percussion elicits sounds that give clues to the makeup of the underlying tissue.

Direct percussion
Using one or two fingers, tap directly on the body part. Ask the patient to tell you which areas are painful, and watch his face for signs of discomfort. This technique is often used to assess an adult patient's sinuses for tenderness, as shown below.

Indirect percussion
Press the distal part of the middle finger of your nondominant hand firmly on the body part. Keep the rest of your hand off the body surface. Flex the wrist, but not the forearm, of your dominant hand. Using the middle finger of your dominant hand, tap quickly and directly over the point where your other middle finger contacts the patient's skin, keeping the fingers perpendicular. Listen to the sounds produced.

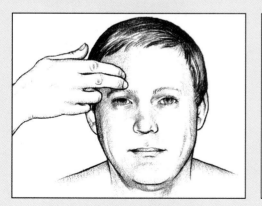

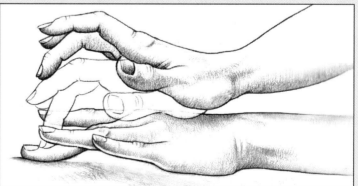

you to locate organ borders, identify organ shape and position, and determine if an organ is solid or filled with fluid or gas.

Skilled touch and a trained ear

Percussion requires a skilled touch and an ear trained to detect slight sound variations. (See *Sounds and their sources*.) Organs and tissues produce sounds of varying loudness, pitch, and duration, depending on their density. For instance, air-filled cavities such as the lungs produce markedly different sounds than the liver and other dense tissues.

As you percuss, move gradually from areas of resonance to those of dullness and then compare sounds. Also compare sounds on one side of the body to sounds on the other side.

Auscultation

Auscultation, usually the last step, involves listening for various breath, heart, and bowel sounds with a stethoscope. (See *Using a stethoscope*.) Because your stethoscope touches many people, be sure to clean the heads and end pieces with alcohol or a disinfectant to prevent the spread of infection.

What does it all mean?

Sounds and their sources

As you practice percussion, you'll recognize different sounds. Each sound is related to the structure underneath. This chart offers a quick guide to percussion sounds and their sources.

Sound	Quality of sound	Where it's heard	Source
Tympany	Drumlike sound	Over enclosed air	Puffed-out cheek; air in bowel
Resonance	Hollow sound	Over areas of part air and part solid	Normal lung
Hyperresonance	Booming sound	Over air	Lung with emphysema
Dullness	Thudlike sound	Over solid tissue	Liver, spleen, heart
Flatness	Flat sound	Over dense tissue	Muscle, bone

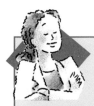

Peak technique

Using a stethoscope

Even if using a stethoscope is second nature to you, it might still be a good idea to brush up on your technique. For starters, your stethoscope should have these features:
• snug-fitting ear plugs, which you'll position toward your nose
• tubing no longer than 15″ (38 cm) and an internal diameter not greater than ⅛″ (0.3 cm)
• a diaphragm and a bell.

How to auscultate
Hold the diaphragm firmly enough against the patient's skin to leave a slight ring afterward. Hold the bell lightly against the skin, just enough to form a seal. Holding the bell too firmly causes the skin to act as a diaphragm, obliterating low-pitched sounds.

Hair on the chest may cause friction on the endpiece, which can mimic abnormal breath sounds such as crackles. You can minimize this problem by lightly wetting the hair before auscultating.

A few more tips
Also keep these points in mind:
• Provide a quiet environment.
• Make sure the area to be auscultated is exposed. Don't try to auscultate over a gown or bed linens — they can interfere with sounds.
• Warm the stethoscope head in your hand.
• Close your eyes to help focus your attention.
• Listen to and try to identify the characteristics of one sound at a time.

Memory jogger

Remembering that the bell of a stethoscope is used to hear low-pitched sounds and the diaphragm is used for high-pitched sounds is easy: "Bell" and "low" both contain the letter "l."

Recording your findings

Begin your documentation with general information, including the patient's age, race, sex, general appearance, height, weight, body mass, vital signs, communication skills, behavior, awareness, orientation, and level of cooperation. (See *Documenting your findings*, page 30.)

Next, precisely record all information you obtained using the four physical assessment techniques.

Just as you followed an organized sequence in your examination, so too should you follow an organized pattern for recording your findings. Document all information about one body system, for example, before proceeding to another.

Documenting your findings

Whether documenting an initial assessment on a patient admitted to your unit or writing a routine assessment note after a home visit, you will need to document your findings using the appropriate form. The illustration below is an example of part of an initial assessment form similar to one you might use.

GENERAL INFORMATION

Age _55_   Sex _M_   Height _163 cm (5'4")_   Weight _51 kg (126 lbs)_

T _37°C (98.6°F)_   P _16_   R _14_   B/P(R) _150/90 sitting_   **(L)** _____

Room _328_

Admission time _0800_

Admission date _8-26-91_

Doctor _Hardy_

Admitting diagnosis

___ _Pneumonia_ ___

Patient's stated reason for

hospitalization _To get_

rid of the pneumonia.

Allergies _None_

Current medications _None_

Name	Dosage	Last taken

GENERAL SURVEY

___ In no acute distress, slender, appears younger than stated age. Is alert ___
___ and well-groomed. Communicates well. Makes eye contact and expresses ___
___ appropriate concern throughout exam. ___

Locate landmarks

Use anatomic landmarks in your descriptions so other people caring for the patient can compare their findings to yours. For instance, you might describe a wound as "1½" × 2½", located 2½" below the umbilicus at the midclavicular line."

With some structures, such as the tympanic membrane or rectum, you can pinpoint a finding by its position on a clock. For instance, you might write "rectal lesion at 3 o'clock." If you use this method, however, make sure others recognize the same landmark for the 12 o'clock reference point.

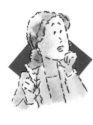

Quick quiz

1. The first technique you'll use in your physical assessment sequence is:
  A. palpation.
  B. auscultation.
  C. inspection.

Answer: C. The assessment of each body system begins with inspection. The most frequently used technique, inspection can reveal more than the other techniques.

2. When palpating the abdomen, begin by palpating:
  A. lightly
  B. firmly.
  C. deeply.

Answer: A. Light palpation is always done first to detect surface characteristics.

3. If you're auscultating the lungs of a man with chest hair:
  A. shave the chest first.
  B. lightly wet the hair
  C. use the diaphragm instead of the bell.

Answer: B. Lightly wet the hair to prevent friction on the endpiece of the stethoscope, which can mimic abnormal breath sounds.

4. A diastolic blood pressure reading reflects:
  A. minimum systemic arterial pressure during left ventricular relaxation.
  B. minimum systemic arterial pressure during left ventricular contraction.
  C. minimum systemic arterial pressure between left ventricular contraction and relaxation.

Answer: A. The diastolic blood pressure reflects the minimum systemic arterial pressure that occurs during left ventricular relaxation. This reading is often a more important indicator of cardiac functions than the systolic blood pressure.

5. The pulse deficit measures the difference between the:

    A. apical and radial pulse rates.

    B. systolic and diastolic blood pressure.

    C. systolic blood pressure and atrial pulse rate.

Answer: A. The pulse deficit is the difference between the apical rate and the radial rate. It provides an indirect evaluation of the ability of each heart contraction to eject enough blood into the peripheral circulation.

6. You're performing percussion on a patient and you hear a flat sound. The most likely source of this sound is:

    A. normal tissue.

    B. lung with emphysema.

    C. muscle.

Answer: C. Flatness is most commonly heard over dense tissue, such as muscle or bone.

Scoring

☆☆☆ If you answered all six items correctly, hooray! You're a history-takin', physical-assessin', proudly-palpatin' assessment whiz!

☆☆ If you answered four or five correctly, terrific! You're a hands-on winner!

☆ If you answered fewer than four correctly, that's okay! In our assessment, you've got great potential!

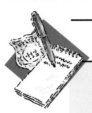

③

Nutritional assessment

Just the facts

This chapter explains how to assess your patient's nutritional status. In this chapter, you'll learn:

♦ about the importance of nutrition to health

♦ what questions about nutrition to ask your patient during the health history

♦ how to assess body systems as part of a nutritional assessment

♦ how to take anthropometric measurements

♦ what laboratory tests help diagnose nutritional problems

♦ what abnormalities you may discover during a nutritional assessment.

A look at nutritional assessment

A patient's nutritional health can influence his body's response to illness and treatment. Regardless of your patient's overall condition, evaluating his nutritional health should be a critical part of your total assessment. (See *Parts of a nutritional assessment,* page 34.) A better understanding of your patient's nutritional status can help you plan his care more effectively.

Normal nutrition

Nutrition refers to the sum of the processes by which a living organism ingests, digests, absorbs, transports, uses, and excretes nutrients. For nutrition to be adequate, a person must receive the proper nutrients, including proteins, fats, carbohydrates, water, vitamins, and minerals. In addition, his digestive system must function properly for his body to make use of nutrients.

Break it down

The body breaks down nutrients mechanically and chemically into simpler compounds for absorption in the stomach and intestines. The mechanical breakdown of food begins with chewing and then continues in the stomach and intestine as food is churned in the GI tract. The chemical processes start with the salivary enzymes in the mouth and continue with acid and enzyme action throughout the rest of the GI tract.

Use it now... or later

Nutrients can be used for the body's immediate needs, or they can be stored for later use. (See *Anabolism and catabolism.*) For example, glucose, a carbohydrate, is stored in muscle and the liver. It can be converted quickly when the body needs energy fast. If glucose isn't available, the body breaks down stored fat, a source of energy during periods of starvation.

Protein power

The body needs protein for normal growth and function and to maintain body tissues. Protein is stored in muscle, bone, blood, skin, cartilage, and lymph and is broken down by the body as a source of energy when the supply of carbohydrates and fat is inadequate. Vitamins, minerals, and water are also essential for normal functioning of the body.

Lipids on the loose

Lipids and other fats are also essential for normal functioning. In order to be transported throughout the body, lipids combine with plasma proteins to form lipoproteins. Likewise, free fatty acids combine with albumin, and cholesterol, triglycerides, and phospholipids bind to globulin.

Parts of a nutritional assessment

Remember the four parts of a nutritional assessment, shown here.

HEALTH HISTORY   LABORATORY TESTS

BODY SYSTEMS ASSESSMENT   ANTHROPOMETRIC MEASUREMENTS

Obtaining a nutritional health history

The first step in a nutritional assessment is the health history. Patients may come to you with a variety of nutrition-related complaints. They may complain of weight gain or loss; changes in their energy level, appetite, or taste; dysphagia; GI tract problems, such as nausea or diarrhea; or other body system changes, such as skin or nail abnormalities. Investigate those complaints as you would any other chief complaint.

During your interview, ask the patient about previous medical problems, current medications, unusual physical activity, intentional weight loss or gain, allergies, smoking, eating patterns, alcohol or drug use, food choices, and vitamin use. Also ask about a family history of obesity, diabetes, metabolic disorders such as hypercholesterolemia, or stomach and GI disturbances. These problems commonly recur in families.

A day in the life

In addition, ask the patient to describe his typical day. This will give you important information about his routine activity level and eating habits. Ask him to recount what and how much he ate yesterday, how the food was cooked, and who cooked it.

Besides telling you about the patient's usual food intake, this information gives clues about food preferences, eating patterns, and even the patient's memory and mental status. (See *Understanding differences in food intake*, page 36.)

Performing the assessment

After completing the health history, you'll perform a two-part nutritional physical assessment. In part one, you'll assess several key body systems. In part two, you'll take anthropometric measurements. Remember that nutritional problems may be associated with various disorders or factors. (See *Tips for detecting nutritional problems*, page 37.)

Anabolism and catabolism

Anabolism is a "building up" process that occurs when simple substances, such as nutrients, are converted into more complex compounds to be used for tissue growth, maintenance, and repair.

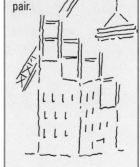

Catabolism is a "breaking down" process that occurs when complex substances are converted into simple compounds and stored or used for energy.

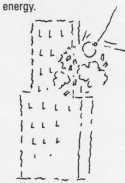

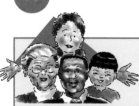

Understanding differences in food intake

What your patient eats depends on a variety of cultural and economic influences. Understanding these influences will give you more insight into the patient's nutritional status.

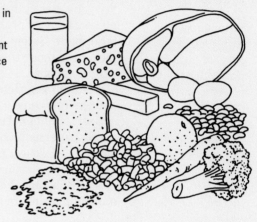

• *Socioeconomic status* may affect a patient's ability to afford healthful foods in the quantities needed to maintain proper health. Low socioeconomic status can lead to nutritional problems, especially for small children and for pregnant women, who may give birth to infants with low birth weight or may experience complications of labor.

• *Work schedule* can affect the amount and type of food a patient eats, especially if he works full-time at night.

• *Religion* can restrict food choices. For instance, observant Jews and Muslims don't eat pork products, and Catholics avoid meat on Ash Wednesday and Fridays during Lent.

• *Ethnic background* influences food choices. For example, fish and rice are staple foods for many Asian people.

Take a good look

Before starting your physical assessment, quickly evaluate the patient's general appearance. Does he look rested? Is his posture good? Are his height and weight in proportion to his body build? Are his physical movements smooth with no apparent weaknesses? Is he free of skeletal deformities?

Assessing each body system

Next, do a head-to-toe assessment of the patient's major body systems. In addition to observing the patient's body structure, you'll want to include the following areas in your assessment.

Skin, hair, and nails

When assessing the patient's skin, hair, and nails, ask yourself these questions: Is his hair shiny and full? Is his skin free of blemishes or rashes? Is it warm and dry, with normal color for that particular patient? Are his nails firm with pink beds?

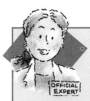

Advice from the experts

Tips for detecting nutritional problems

Nutritional problems may stem from physical conditions, drugs, diet, or lifestyle factors. The checklist below will help you find out if your patient is a likely candidate for a nutritional problem.

Physical condition
- Chronic illnesses, such as diabetes or neurologic, cardiac, or thyroid problems
- Family history of diabetes or heart disease
- Draining wounds or fistulas
- Obesity or a weight gain of 20% above normal body weight
- Unplanned weight loss of 20% below normal body weight
- History of or recent GI disturbances
- Anorexia or bulimia
- Depression or anxiety
- Severe trauma
- Recent chemotherapy or radiation therapy
- Physical limitations, such as paresis or paralysis
- Recent major surgery
- Pregnancy, especially teen or multiple-birth pregnancy

Drugs and diet
- Fad diets
- Steroid, diuretic, or antacid use
- Mouth, tooth, or denture problems
- Excessive alcohol intake
- Strict vegetarian diet
- Liquid diet or nothing by mouth for more than 3 days

Lifestyle factors
- Lack of support from family or friends
- Financial problems

Eyes, nose, throat, and neck

Are the patient's eyes clear and shiny? Are the mucous membranes in his nose moist and pink? Is his tongue pink with papillae present? Are his gums moist and pink? Is his mouth free of ulcers or lesions? Is his neck free of masses that would impede swallowing?

Cardiovascular system

Is the patient's heart rhythm regular? Are his heart rate and blood pressure normal for his age? Are his extremities free of swelling?

GI system

Is the patient's appetite satisfactory, with no reported GI problems? Are his elimination patterns regular? Is his abdomen free of abnormal masses on palpation?

Neurologic system

Is the patient alert and responsive? Are his reflexes normal, and is his behavior appropriate? Are his legs and feet free of paresthesia?

Anthropometric measurements

The second part of the physical assessment is taking anthropometric measurements. These measurements can help identify nutritional problems, especially in patients who are seriously overweight or underweight. You won't always need to perform all measurements. Let the results of the patient's health history guide you. Two important anthropometric measurements are height and weight.

Measuring height and weight

If your patient can stand without assistance, measure his height using the height bar on a scale. If he's weak or bedridden, use a measuring stick or tape. (See *Overcoming problems in measuring height.*) Weigh the mobile patient using a calibrated balance beam scale. Use a bed scale for a bedridden patient.

That elusive ideal weight

You've probably heard the term ideal body weight, a term that refers to standard weights associated with various heights on a reference table. (See *Height and weight table.*) Weight as a percentage of ideal body weight is obtained by dividing the patient's true weight by his ideal body weight—a number found on a table—and then multiplying that number by 100.

A body weight of 120% or more of ideal body weight indicates obesity. Below 90% indicates less than adequate weight.

Anthropometric alternatives

Other anthropometric measurements include midarm circumference, midarm muscle circumference, and skinfold thickness. (See *Taking anthropometric arm measurements*, page 40.) Those measurements are used to evaluate muscle mass and subcutaneous fat, both of which relate to nutritional status.

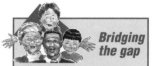

Bridging the gap

Overcoming problems in measuring height

Do you need to measure your patient's height but he is confined to a wheelchair? Or is he unable to stand straight because of scoliosis? You can still get an approximate measurement of his height using the "wingspan" technique.

Have the patient hold his arms straight out from the sides of his body. Tell children to hold their arms out "like bird wings." Then measure from the tip of one middle finger to the tip of the other. That distance is the patient's approximate height.

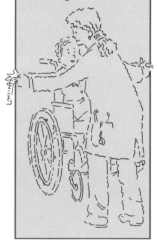

Height and weight table

Ongoing research suggests that people can carry a bit more weight as they age without added health risk. Because people of the same height may differ in muscle and bone makeup, a range of weights is shown for each height in the table below. The higher weights in each category apply to men, who typically have more muscle and bone than women. Height measurements are without shoes; weight measurements are without clothes.

Height	Weight	
	Ages 19 to 34	Ages 35 and over
5'0"	97 to 128	108 to 138
5'1"	101 to 132	111 to 143
5'2"	104 to 137	115 to 148
5'3"	107 to 141	119 to 152
5'4"	111 to 146	122 to 157
5'5"	114 to 150	126 to 162
5'6"	118 to 155	130 to 167
5'7"	121 to 160	134 to 172
5'8"	125 to 164	138 to 178
5'9"	129 to 169	142 to 183
5'10"	132 to 174	146 to 188
5'11"	136 to 179	151 to 194
6'0"	140 to 184	155 to 199
6'1"	144 to 189	159 to 205
6'2"	148 to 195	164 to 210
6'3"	152 to 200	168 to 216
6'4"	156 to 205	172 to 222
6'5"	160 to 211	177 to 228
6'6"	164 to 216	182 to 234

Weighty terms

Here are some weight-related definitions:
• normal weight: 10% above or below recommended weight
• overweight: 10% to 20% above recommended weight
• obese: 20% or more above recommended weight
• underweight: 10% to 20% below recommended weight

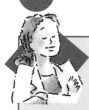

Peak technique

Taking anthropometric arm measurements

Follow these steps to determine the triceps' skin-fold thickness, midarm circumference, and midarm muscle circumference.

Triceps' skin-fold thickness

1. Find the midpoint circumference of the arm by placing the tape measure halfway between the axilla and the elbow. Grasp the patient's skin with your thumb and forefinger, about ⅓″ (1 cm) above the midpoint, as shown.

2. Place calipers at the midpoint and squeeze for 3 seconds.

3. Record the measurement to the nearest millimeter.

4. Take two more readings and use the average.

Midarm circumference and midarm muscle circumference

1. At the midpoint, measure the midarm circumference, as shown. Record the measurement in centimeters.

2. Calculate the midarm muscle circumference by multiplying the triceps' skinfold thickness — measured in millimeters — by 3.14.

3. Subtract this number from the midarm circumference.

Recording the measurements

Record all three measurements as a percentage of the standard measurements (see chart below), using this formula:

$$\frac{\text{Actual measurement}}{\text{Standard measurement}} \times 100 = \%$$

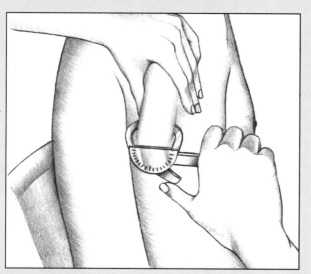

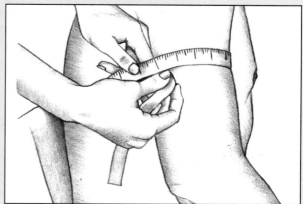

After you've taken all the measurements, apply these rules:
- A measurement less than 90% of the standard indicates caloric deprivation.
- A measurement over 90% indicates adequate or more than adequate energy reserves.

Measurement	Standard	90%
Triceps' skin-fold thickness	Men: 12.5 mm Women: 16.5 mm	Men: 11.3 mm Women: 14.9 mm
Midarm circumference	Men: 29.3 cm Women: 28.5 cm	Men: 26.4 cm Women: 25.7cm
Midarm muscle circumference	Men: 25.3 cm Women: 23.3 cm	Men: 22.8 cm Women: 20.9 cm

• seriously underweight: 20% or more below recommended weight.

Laboratory studies

The last part of the nutritional assessment is an evaluation of the patient's laboratory test results. Here are some common biochemical tests done as part of a nutritional assessment and what the results of those tests might mean. Other tests, such as thyroid function tests and serum electrolyte and vitamin levels, may also be ordered.

All about albumin

The serum albumin level assesses protein levels in the body. Albumin makes up more than 50% of total proteins in the serum and affects the cardiovascular system because it helps maintain plasma osmotic pressure. Keep in mind that albumin production requires functioning liver cells and an adequate supply of amino acids, the building blocks of proteins.

The serum albumin level is decreased with serious protein deficiency and loss of blood protein due to burns, malnutrition, liver or renal disease, congestive heart failure, major surgery, infections, or cancer.

Here's to hemoglobin!

Hemoglobin is the main component of red blood cells, which transport oxygen. Its formation requires an adequate supply of protein in the form of amino acids. Hemoglobin values help assess the oxygen-carrying capacity of the blood and are useful in diagnosing anemia, protein deficiency, and hydration status.

A decreased hemoglobin suggests iron deficiency anemia, protein deficiency, excessive blood loss, or overhydration. An increased hemoglobin suggests dehydration or polycythemia.

Don't omit hematocrit

The hematocrit level reflects the proportion of blood occupied by red blood cells. This test helps diagnose anemia and dehydration. Decreased values suggest iron-deficiency anemia or excessive fluid intake or blood loss. Increased values suggest severe dehydration or polycythemia.

Carry on with transferrin

Transferrin is a "carrier" protein that transports iron. The molecule is synthesized mainly in the liver. A serum transferrin level reflects the patient's current protein status more accurately than albumin because of its shorter half-life. The level decreases along with protein levels and indicates depletion of protein stores.

Decreased values may also indicate inadequate protein production due to liver damage, protein loss from renal disease, acute or chronic infection, or cancer. Elevated levels may indicate severe iron deficiency.

Next comes nitrogen

A nitrogen balance test involves collecting all urine during a 24-hour period to determine how well protein is being used by the body. Proteins contain nitrogen, and when they're broken down into amino acids, nitrogen is excreted in the urine as urea.

Nitrogen intake and excretion should be equal. The nitrogen balance is the difference between nitrogen intake and excretion. It's calculated using a formula, and the results are interpreted to determine whether the patient is receiving enough, too much, or not enough protein. Results may vary with such conditions as burns and infection.

Check out the creatinine height index

The test for creatinine height index involves a 24-hour urine collection to measure urinary excretion of creatinine. It helps define body protein mass and evaluate protein depletion. Test results are interpreted using a formula that compares results to ideal height standards.

Values decrease with age because of the decrease in lean muscle mass. The test is of limited value because results are greatly altered by age, amount of exercise, stress, menstruation, and the presence of a severe illness. Increased values may indicate decreased protein stores.

Total the lymphocytes

The total lymphocyte count evaluates the health of the immune system and assists in the evaluation of protein stores. Decreased values may indicate malnutrition when no other cause is apparent. They may also point to infection, leukemia, or tissue necrosis.

Trust in triglycerides

Triglycerides are the main storage form of lipids. Measuring triglyceride levels can help identify early hyperlipemia. However, increased levels alone aren't diagnostic; further studies are required such as cholesterol measurement. Decreased levels of triglycerides occur in malnutrition.

Count the cholesterol

A total cholesterol test measures circulating levels of free cholesterol and cholesterol esters. A diet high in saturated fats raises cholesterol levels by stimulating lipid absorption. Increased levels indicate an increased risk of coronary artery disease. Decreased levels are commonly associated with malnutrition.

Nutritional disorders

Patients with nutritional problems generally have one of the following disorders: protein-calorie malnutrition, obesity, anorexia nervosa, bulimia, or a vitamin deficiency. Be aware that patients hospitalized for more than 2 weeks are at risk for nutritional disorders.

Protein-calorie malnutrition

Protein-calorie, or protein-energy, malnutrition is a term given to a spectrum of disorders caused by either prolonged or chronic inadequate protein or calorie intake or by high metabolic protein and energy requirements. When protein or calorie intake is inadequate, the body meets its energy needs by breaking down and using stored proteins and fats.

Three major disorders fall under the heading of protein-calorie malnutrition: marasmus, kwashiorkor, and marasmus-kwashiorkor mix.

Marasmus

Marasmus, or protein-calorie malnutrition, occurs primarily in children 6 to 18 months old and results from a chronic lack of nutrients. (See *Detecting marasmus*.) It impairs brain development and causes failure to thrive. It may also occur in patients with anorexia, starvation, bowel obstruction, and chronic illness.

Detecting marasmus

In marasmus, the patient starves from prolonged lack of calories, protein, and nearly all other nutrients. The illness usually occurs in infants living in poverty, but it may also strike the elderly poor or young adults who have dieted excessively.

Diagnostic test results reveal vitamin and mineral deficiencies. With treatment, the patient has a fair prognosis.

Signs of marasmus
Marasmus may lead to the following signs and symptoms:

- emaciated appearance
- muscle wasting
- loss of subcutaneous fat
- subnormal body temperature
- decreased resistance to infection
- failure to thrive in infants or the elderly
- hair loss
- dry, atrophic, loose skin, especially around the thighs and buttocks
- mental and physical growth retardation in infants and children.

Detecting kwashiorkor

A severe protein deficiency, kwashiorkor results from insufficient intake of quality protein. It's usually associated with adequate or even excessive calorie intake or with a high-carbohydrate diet, and it typically accompanies an acute illness. Diagnostic test results show vitamin and mineral deficiencies (especially vitamins A and B), anemia, and low serum albumin, potassium, lymphocyte, and transferrin levels.

Left untreated, kwashiorkor causes death in most instances. With treatment, however, the patient's prognosis is good.

Look for these signs
People with kwashiorkor typically suffer from:

- generalized illness, possibly involving fever
- weight loss and muscle wasting, possibly masked by facial edema or edema in the lower body, producing a potbelly
- sparse, thin, soft hair, possibly with parallel gray, red, or blond streaks
- changes in the mucous membranes, including cracks at the corners of the mouth, mouth ulcerations and lesions, and tongue atrophy
- scaly skin, dermatosis, and reddish skin and hair pigmentation
- enlarged liver
- apathy and irritability
- poor appetite
- anorexia
- diarrhea
- reduced resistance to infection
- poor wound healing.

Although blood and visceral protein levels may be normal, skeletal muscle wasting and loss of subcutaneous fat occurs. Skin-fold and midarm muscle circumference measurements are smaller than normal, and the patient looks emaciated.

Kwashiorkor

Kwashiorkor, or protein malnutrition, occurs in young children, usually when they're weaned from breast-feeding after the birth of a sibling. (See *Detecting kwashiorkor*.) Anthropometric measurements may be normal. Children may even appear obese, but a loss of visceral protein occurs.

Low-protein diets, fad diets, and the prolonged use of I.V. dextrose can cause kwashiorkor. Edema, lack of pigmentation in the skin and hair, and depressed immune function may occur as well as decreased serum albumin and transferrin levels.

Marasmus-kwashiorkor mix

Marasmus-kwashiorkor mix affects chronically starved people subjected to acute distress. It causes a loss of subcutaneous fat, immune system damage, and depletion of blood, visceral, and muscle protein. Of the three types of malnutrition, this is the most serious and is associated with starvation, burns, and trauma.

Obesity

Obesity is defined as weight more than 20% above ideal body weight and is due to an imbalance of calorie intake and calorie use. Although an obese patient consumes more than adequate food quantities, he may still be malnourished and have deficiencies in certain nutrients as a result of eating an imbalanced diet. Causes of obesity are varied. Immune function is usually normal, and anthropometric measurements are increased.

Anorexia nervosa

A psychosocial disorder, anorexia nervosa is an intentional loss of at least 25% of body weight. Physical signs include muscle wasting; fat store depletion; dry, inelastic skin; loss or change in hair; constipation; amenorrhea; hypotension; and bradycardia. You may also find loss of tooth enamel because of prolonged vomiting.

Bulimia

Bulimia, a binge-purge syndrome, is more deceptive than anorexia nervosa because the patient typically has normal or above-normal body weight or frequent fluctuations in weight. (See *Evaluating nutritional disorders,* page 46.) Weight is controlled by the use of vomiting, emetics, laxatives, diuretics, and diet pills. Electrolyte imbalances, gum infections, and loss of tooth enamel may occur.

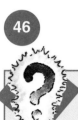

What does it all mean?

Evaluating nutritional disorders

Quickly scan this chart to help you interpret your nutritional assessment findings.

Body system or region	Sign or symptom	Implications
General	• Weakness, fatigue • Weight loss	• Anemia, electrolyte imbalance • Decreased calorie intake or increased calorie use, inadequate nutrient intake or absorption
Skin, hair, nails	• Dry, flaky skin • Dry skin with poor turgor • Rough scaly skin with bumps • Petechiae or ecchymoses • Sore that won't heal • Thinning, dry hair • Spoon-shaped, brittle, or ridged nails	• Vitamin A, vitamin B-complex, or linoleic acid deficiency • Dehydration • Vitamin A deficiency • Vitamin C or K deficiency • Protein, vitamin C, or zinc deficiency • Protein deficiency • Iron deficiency
Eyes	• Night blindness; corneal swelling, softening, or dryness; Bitot's spots (gray triangular patches on the conjunctiva) • Red conjunctiva	• Vitamin A deficiency • Riboflavin deficiency
Throat, mouth	• Cracks at corner of mouth • Magenta tongue • Beefy, red tongue • Soft, spongy, bleeding gums • Swollen neck (goiter)	• Riboflavin or niacin deficiency • Riboflavin deficiency • Vitamin B_{12} deficiency • Vitamin C deficiency • Iodine deficiency
Cardiovascular	• Edema • Tachycardia, hypotension	• Protein deficiency • Fluid volume deficit
Gastrointestinal	• Ascites	• Protein deficiency
Musculoskeletal	• Bone pain, bow leg • Muscle wasting	• Vitamin D or calcium deficiency • Protein, carbohydrate, and fat deficiency
Neurologic	• Altered mental status • Paresthesia	• Dehydration; thiamine, or vitamin B_{12} deficiency • Vitamin B_{12}, pyridoxine, or thiamine deficiency

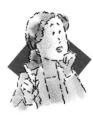

Quick quiz

1. Measuring a patient's midarm circumference is done whenever you:
    A. conduct a basic nutritional assessment.
    B. want to confirm an abnormal protein level.
    C. suspect a serious nutritional problem.

Answer: C. Measuring midarm circumference isn't done unless you suspect a serious nutritional problem.

2. A serum albumin test assesses:
    A. protein levels in the body.
    B. the ratio of protein to albumin.
    C. how well the liver metabolizes proteins.

Answer: A. Albumin makes up more than 50% of total proteins in the serum. The test assesses protein levels in the body.

3. The term nitrogen balance refers to the difference between:
    A. nitrogen intake and stores.
    B. nitrogen intake and excretion.
    C. nitrogen stores and excretion.

Answer: B. The term nitrogen balance refers to the difference between nitrogen intake and excretion. It's calculated using a formula and should indicate that nitrogen intake and excretion are equal.

4. During a nutritional assessment, a patient's lymphocyte count helps to assess for:
    A. bleeding disorders.
    B. cardiovascular function.
    C. severity of malnutrition.

Answer: C. The lymphocyte count, which decreases with malnutrition, evaluates immune system integrity and helps evaluate protein stores.

5. Marasmus occurs primarily in:
    A. infants ages 6 to 18 months.
    B. children ages 2 to 6 years.
    C. children ages 10 to 13 years.

Answer: A. Marasmus, or protein-calorie malnutrition, occurs primarily in infants ages 6 to 18 months and results from a chronic lack of nutrients.

6. Catabolism is defined as a:
   A. process whereby complex substances are converted into simple compounds and stored or used for energy.
   B. process whereby simple substances are converted into complex compounds used to grow and maintain tissues.
   C. primitive practice whereby a member of an enemy tribe or an unsuspecting tourist is roasted for dinner (also called *cannibalism*).

Answer. A. Catabolism is a "breaking down" process in which complex substances are converted into simple compounds and stored or used for energy.

Scoring

☆☆☆ If you answered all six items correctly, congratulations! Reward yourself with dinner and champagne at an elegant restaurant!

☆☆ If you answered four or five correctly, way to go! Treat yourself to a steak and brew at your favorite neighborhood restaurant!

☆ If you answered fewer than four correctly, no sweat. You deserve a break at your favorite pizza or fast-food hot spot!

Part II

Assessing body systems

Skin, hair, and nails

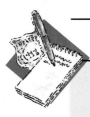

Just the facts

This chapter describes how to assess a patient's skin, hair, and nails. In this chapter, you'll learn:

♦ what skin, hair, and nails consist of

♦ how to distinguish changes in skin, hair, and nails that are normal outcomes of aging from changes that signal a health problem

♦ what questions to ask about skin, hair, and nails during the health history

♦ how to use inspection and palpation to assess skin, hair, and nails

♦ how to identify disorders of the skin, hair, and nails.

A look at skin, hair, and nails

The skin covers the internal structures of the body and protects them from the external world. Along with hair and nails, the skin provides a window for viewing changes taking place inside the body. As a nurse, you observe a patient's skin, hair, and nails regularly, so you'll often detect abnormalities first. Your sharp assessment skills will help supply a reliable picture of the patient's overall health.

To perform an accurate physical assessment, you'll need to understand the anatomy and physiology of the skin, hair, and nails. Let's take them one by one.

Skin

Also called the integumentary system, the skin is the body's largest organ and has several important functions, including:

• protecting underlying tissues from trauma, bacteria, and other harmful agents
• sensing temperature, pain, touch, and pressure
• regulating body temperature through sweat production and evaporation
• synthesizing vitamin D.

Layers of the skin

The skin consists of two distinct layers: the epidermis and the dermis. (See *What's in your skin*.) Subcutaneous tissue lies beneath these layers.

What's in your skin

This cross section of the skin illustrates major skin structures.

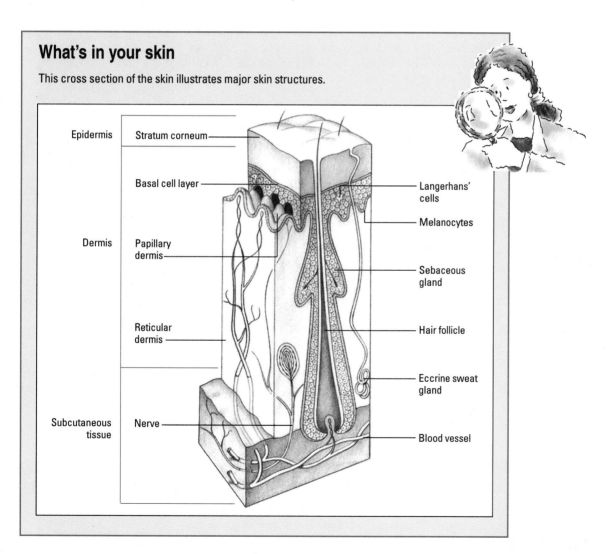

Epidermis — Stratum corneum

Basal cell layer

Langerhans' cells

Melanocytes

Dermis — Papillary dermis

Sebaceous gland

Reticular dermis

Hair follicle

Eccrine sweat gland

Subcutaneous tissue — Nerve

Blood vessel

The epidermis—the outer layer—is made of squamous epithelial tissue. The two major layers of the epidermis are the stratum corneum—the most superficial layer—and the deeper basal cell layer.

Migrating to the outer surface

The stratum corneum is comprised of cells that form in the basal cell layer and migrate to the outer surface of the skin. These cells die as they reach the surface. New cells are constantly being produced, however, because epidermal regeneration is continuous.

The basal cell layer contains melanocytes, which produce melanin and are responsible for skin color.

Melanocyte production is influenced by hormones, the environment, and heredity. Production is greater in some people than in others, hence the wide variation in skin color.

Laying it on thick

The dermis—the thick, deeper layer—consists of connective tissue and an extracellular material called matrix, which contributes to the skin's strength and pliability. Blood vessels, lymphatic vessels, nerves, and hair follicles are located in the dermis, as are sweat and sebaceous glands. Wound healing and infection control take place in the dermis.

Give the glands a hand!

Sebaceous glands, found primarily in the skin of the scalp, face, upper body, and anogenital region, are part of the same structure that contains the hair follicles. Their main function is to produce sebum, which is secreted onto the skin or into the hair follicle to make the hair shiny and pliant.

Apocrine and eccrine glands, or sweat glands, secrete a watery fluid that helps regulate body temperature. Apocrine glands are located mainly in the axillae and anogenital areas. Eccrine glands are distributed over most of the body.

Increasing age, declining skin

As people age, all skin functions decline and normal skin changes occur as a result. (See *How skin ages*.) Because of that decline, elderly patients are more prone to skin disease, infection, problems in wound healing, and tissue atrophy.

Hair

Hair is formed from keratin and produced by matrix cells in the dermal layer. (See *A closer look at hair*, page 54.)

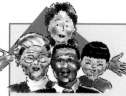

Bridging the gap

How skin ages

The table below lists skin changes that normally occur with aging.

Change	Finding
Pigmentation	• Pale skin color
Thickness	• Wrinkling, especially on the face, arms, and legs • Parchmentlike appearance, especially over bony prominences and on the dorsal surfaces of the hands, feet, arms, and legs
Moisture	• Dry, flaky, and rough
Turgor	• Skin "tents" and stands alone
Texture	• Numerous creases and lines • Wrinkling, especially around the eyes and face

Each hair lies in a hair follicle and receives nourishment from the papilla, a loop of capillaries at the base of the follicle. At the lower end of the hair shaft is the hair bulb, which contains melanocytes that determine hair color.

Each hair is attached at the base to a smooth muscle called the arrector pili. This muscle contracts during emotional stress or exposure to cold and elevates the hair, causing "goose flesh."

Hair today, gone tomorrow

The aging process causes many changes in the hair. Melanocyte function declines, producing light or gray hair, and the hair follicle itself becomes drier as sebaceous gland function decreases. Hair growth declines, so the amount of body hair decreases. Balding, genetically determined in younger individuals, occurs in many people as a normal result of aging.

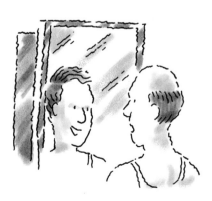

A closer look at hair

The illustration below shows a hair shaft and its associated glands.

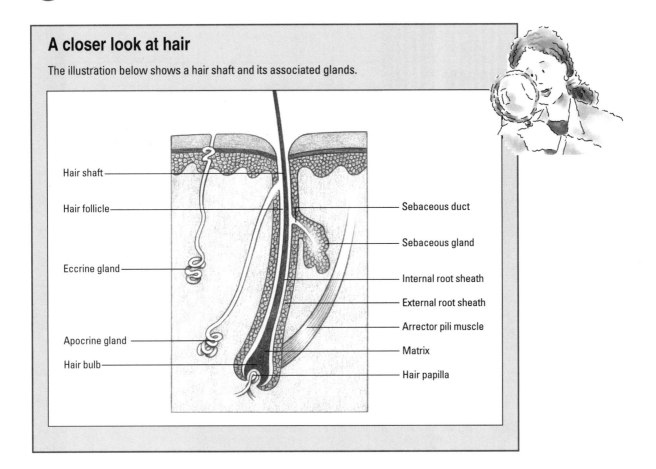

- Hair shaft
- Hair follicle
- Eccrine gland
- Apocrine gland
- Hair bulb
- Sebaceous duct
- Sebaceous gland
- Internal root sheath
- External root sheath
- Arrector pili muscle
- Matrix
- Hair papilla

Nails

Nails are formed when the epidermal cells are converted into hard plates of keratin. (See *Nail anatomy.*) The nails are made up of the nail root (or nail matrix), nail plate, nail bed, lunula, nail folds, and cuticle.

The nail plate is the visible, hardened layer attached to and covering the fingertip. The plate is clear with fine longitudinal ridges. The pink color results from blood vessels underlying vascular epithelial cells.

The nail matrix is the site of nail growth and is protected by the cuticle. At the end of the matrix is the white, crescent-shaped area, the lunula, that extends beyond the cuticle.

Nail anatomy

The illustration below shows the anatomic components of a fingernail.

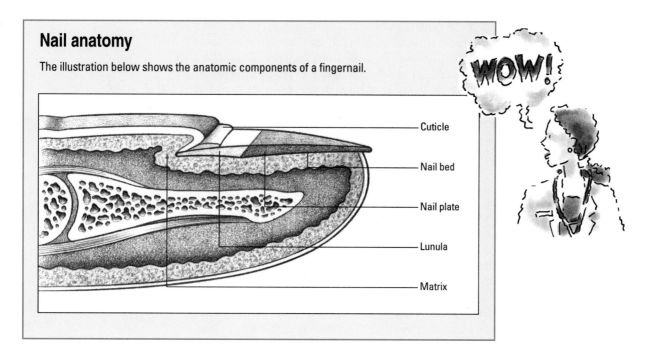

Cuticle

Nail bed

Nail plate

Lunula

Matrix

WOW!

Not hard as nails anymore

With age, nail growth slows and the nails become brittle and thin. Longitudinal ridges in the nail plate become much more pronounced, making the nails prone to splitting. In addition, the nails lose their luster and become yellowed.

Obtaining a health history

When assessing a problem related to skin, hair, or nails, you'll need to thoroughly explore the patient's chief complaint, medical history, family history, psychological history, and patterns of daily living. Keep in mind that skin, hair, and nail abnormalities often arise from a medical problem unrelated to the chief complaint, so they may be overlooked or minimized by the patient.

Asking about the skin

Most chief complaints about the skin involve problems with itching, rashes, lesions, pigmentation abnormalities, or changes in existing lesions.

Typical questions to ask about changes in a patient's skin include: How and when did the skin changes occur? Is there bleeding or drainage from the area? Does the area itch? How much time do you spend in the sun? When spending time in the sun, how do you protect your skin? Do you have allergies? Do you have a family history of cancer or other significant diseases? Do you have a fever, joint pain, or weight loss? Have you recently been bitten by an insect? What medications do you take?

Asking about the hair

Most chief complaints about the hair concern hair loss or increased growth and distribution of body hair, called hirsutism. Either of those problems can be caused by such psychological factors as skin infections, ovarian or adrenal tumors, increased stress, or systemic diseases, such as hypothyroidism or malignancies.

To identify the cause of your patient's hair problem, ask: When did you first notice the loss (or gain) of hair? Was it sudden or gradual? Did the change occur in just a few spots or all over your body? What was happening in your life when the problem started? Are you taking any medications? Are you having itching, pain, discharge, fever, or weight loss? What have you done to treat the problem? Has it helped? What serious illnesses, if any, have you had?

Asking about the nails

The most common complaints about the nails concern changes in growth and color. Infection, nutritional deficiencies, systemic illnesses, and stress can cause those problems.

To gain information about the nails, ask: When did you first notice the changes in your nails? Was it sudden or gradual? Do you have other symptoms, such as bleeding, pain, itching, or discharge? What is the normal condition of your nails? Do you have a history of serious illness? Do you have a history of nail problems? Do you bite your nails? Have you had nail tips attached?

Assessing skin, hair, and nails

To assess skin, hair, and nails, you'll use the techniques of inspection and palpation. Before beginning the examination, make sure the room is well lit and comfortably warm. Wear gloves during your examination.

Skin

Before you begin your skin assessment, gather the following equipment: clear centimeter ruler, tongue depressor, penlight or flashlight, Wood's lamp, and magnifying glass. This equipment will enable you to measure and closely inspect skin lesions and other abnormalities.

Start by observing the overall appearance of the skin. This will help to identify areas that need further assessment. Inspect and palpate the skin area by area, focusing on color, texture, turgor, moisture, and temperature.

Concentrate on skin color

Look for localized areas of bruising, cyanosis, pallor, and erythema. Check for uniformity of color and hypopigmented or hyperpigmented areas. Places exposed to the sun may show a darker pigmentation than other areas. *Remember that color changes may look different in dark-skinned people.* (See *Detecting color variations in dark-skinned people.*)

Target skin texture and turgor

Inspect and palpate the skin's texture, noting its thickness and mobility. It should look smooth and be intact. Rough, dry skin is common in hypothyroidism, psoriasis, and excessive keratinization. Skin that isn't intact may indicate local irritation or trauma.

Palpation will also help you evaluate the patient's state of hydration. Dehydration and edema cause poor skin turgor. (See *Evaluating skin turgor*, page 58.) Overhydration causes the skin to appear edematous and spongy. Localized edema can also result from trauma or systemic disease. *Keep in mind that poor skin turgor also occurs as a normal result of aging, so it may not be a reliable indicator of hydration in the elderly.*

Scrutinize skin moisture

Observe the moisture content of the skin. It should be relatively dry, with a minimal amount of perspiration. Skinfold areas should also be fairly dry. Overly dry skin will look red and flaky. Overly moist skin can be caused by anxiety, obesity, or an environment that's too warm.

Bridging the gap

Detecting color variations in dark-skinned people

Detecting pallor
Examine the sclerae, conjunctiva, buccal mucosa, tongue, lips, nail beds, palms, and soles. Look for an ashen color.

Detecting jaundice
Examine the sclerae and hard palate. Look for a yellow color.

Detecting petechiae
Examine areas of lighter pigmentation, such as the abdomen. Look for tiny, purplish red dots.

Detecting erythema
Palpate the area for warmth.

Detecting edema
Examine the area for decreased color, and palpate for tightness.

Detecting cyanosis
Examine the conjunctiva, palms, soles, buccal mucosa, and tongue. Look for dull, dark color.

Detecting rashes
Palpate the area for skin texture changes.

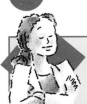

Evaluating skin turgor

To assess skin turgor in an adult, gently squeeze the skin on the forearm or sternal area between your thumb and forefinger, as shown. In an infant, roll a fold of loosely adherent abdominal skin between your thumb and forefinger. Then release the skin.

If the skin quickly returns to its original shape, the patient has normal turgor. If it returns to its original shape slowly over 30 seconds, or maintains a tented position, as shown, the skin has poor turgor.

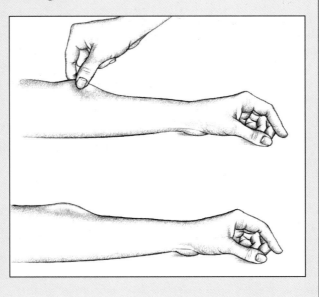

Take stock of skin temperature

Palpate the skin for temperature, which can range from cool to warm. (See *Assessing skin temperature*.) Warm skin suggests normal circulation. Make sure to distinguish between generalized and localized coolness and warmth. Localized skin coolness can result from vasoconstriction associated with cold environments or impaired arterial circulation to a limb. General coolness can result from such conditions as shock or hypothyroidism.

Localized warmth can occur in an area of infection, inflammation, or burn. Generalized warmth occurs with fever or systemic diseases such as hyperthyroidism. Make sure to check skin temperature bilaterally.

Variations in texture and pigmentation

During your inspection, you may see normal variations in the skin's texture and pigmentation. Red, pigmented lesions caused by vascular changes include hemangiomas,

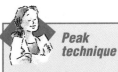

Assessing skin temperature

When you're trying to compare subtle temperature differences in one area of the body to another, use the dorsal surface of your hands and fingers. They're the most sensitive to changes in temperature.

Recognizing common skin disorders

On this page and the pages that follow, you'll find photos of common skin disorders along with brief descriptions of each. Refer to the photos as a guide when assessing abnormal skin findings.

Basal cell carcinoma

The most common skin cancer, basal cell carcinoma results from sun exposure. It's usually a small, waxy-looking nodule that ulcerates and forms a central depression. It rarely metastasizes and commonly appears on the head and neck.

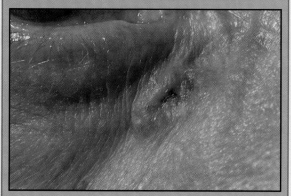

Squamous cell carcinoma

This form of skin cancer results from sun exposure and is able to metastasize. It appears as a raised border with a central ulcer and may appear rough, thickened, or scaly. It appears most often on the face and neck.

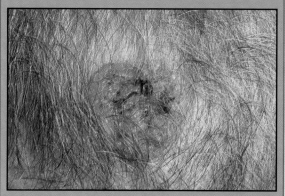

Malignant melanoma

Lesions can occur anywhere on the body and can arise from a preexisting mole. Its border, color, and surface are usually irregular. The color may vary but is usually black or purple, though some lesions are pink, red, or whitish-blue.

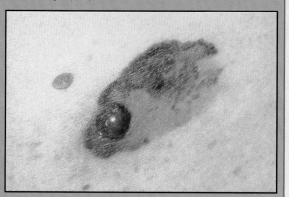

Kaposi's sarcoma

These lesions tend to appear first on the lower legs but they may develop anywhere. Initially, you'll note multiple brown or bluish-red nodules of varying shapes and sizes. The nodules develop into larger plaques. These lesions may open and drain or cause edema of the legs.

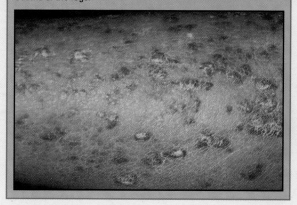

(continued)

Recognizing common skin disorders *(continued)*

Lupus erythematosus (discoid or systemic)

The typical sign of lupus, a butterfly-shaped rash, appears as a red, scaly, sharply demarcated rash over the cheeks and nose. The rash may extend to other areas of the face or other exposed areas, such as the ears or neck.

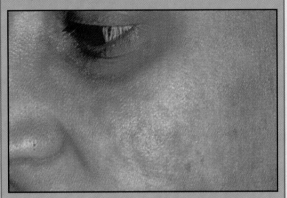

Telangiectasia

Formed by dilation of small blood vessels, telangiectases blanch when pressure is applied, whereas petechiae won't. These lesions may be a normal finding in an elderly person or associated with cirrhosis or lupus.

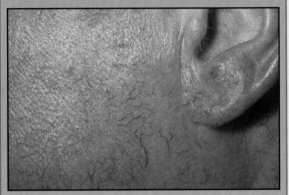

Scabies

Mites picked up from an infested person burrow under the skin and cause scabies lesions. The lesions appear in a straight or a zigzagging line about ⅜" (1 cm) long, with a black dot at the end. Commonly seen between the fingers, at the bend of the elbow and knee, and around the groin or perineal area, scabies lesions itch and may cause a rash.

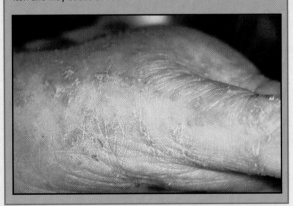

Vitiligo

This slowly progressive disease of hypopigmentation causes irregular areas of pigmented skin around milky patches. The areas commonly appear on the face, hands, and feet.

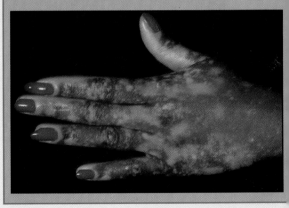

Psoriasis

Psoriasis is a chronic disease of marked epidermal thickening. Plaques are symmetrical and generally appear as a red base topped with silvery scales. The lesions may connect with one another and occur most commonly on the scalp, elbows, and knees.

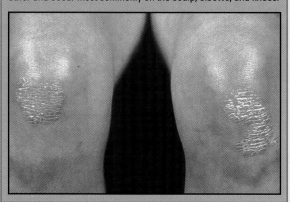

Urticaria (hives)

Occurring as an allergic reaction, this disorder appears suddenly as pink, edematous papules or wheals (round elevations of the skin). Itching is intense. The lesions may become large and contain vesicles.

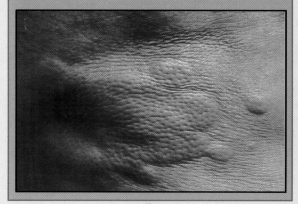

Contact dermatitis

This inflammatory disorder results from contact with an irritant. Primary lesions include vesicles, large oozing bullae, and red macules that appear as localized areas of redness. The lesions may itch and burn.

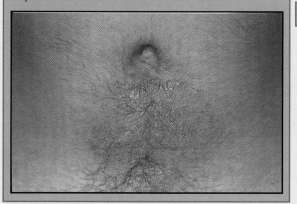

Eczema

This condition may be acute or chronic and accompanied by severe itching. It appears as reddened papules, vesicles, or pustular lesions. It affects mostly the antecubital and popliteal areas. Lesions cause blisters, oozing, and crusting. Thickening, excoriation, and extreme dryness of the skin also occur.

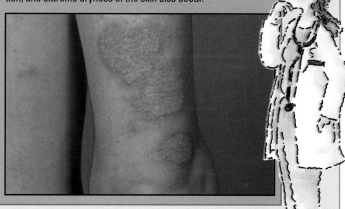

(continued)

Recognizing common skin disorders *(continued)*

Herpes zoster

Herpes zoster appears as grouped vesicles or crusted lesions along a nerve root. The vesicles are usually unilateral and appear mostly on the face, hands, and neck. Lesions cause pain but no itching or rash.

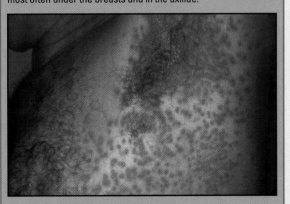

Tinea corporis (ringworm)

These round, red, scaly lesions are accompanied by intense itching. Lesions have slightly raised, red borders consisting of tiny vesicles. Individual rings may connect to form patches with scalloped edges. They usually appear on exposed areas of the body.

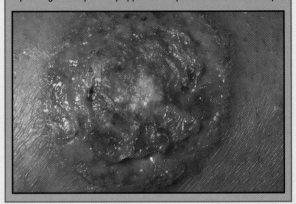

Candidiasis

This fungal infection produces erythema and a scaly papular rash. Because the fungus thrives in moist environments, it occurs most often under the breasts and in the axillae.

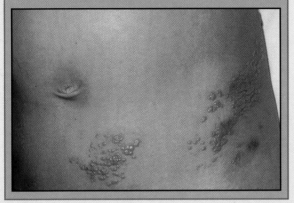

Impetigo

This rash usually appears on the face and is caused by a bacterial infection. When ruptured, fragile vesicles in the rash ooze a honey-colored fluid. Crusts may form.

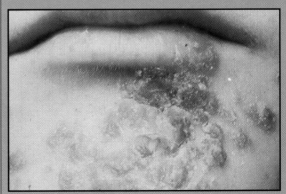

telangiectases, petechiae, purpura, and ecchymoses and may or may not indicate disease.

Other normal variations include birthmarks, freckles, and moles or nevi. Nevi may be pink, tan, or dark brown and either flat or raised. They can be found on all areas of the body. Birthmarks are generally flat and range from tan to red or brown. Like nevi, birthmarks can also be found on any part of the body. Freckles are small, flat macules located primarily on the face, arms, and back. They're usually red-brown to brown.

Where did the lesion come from?

Whenever you see a lesion, evaluate it to determine its origin. Start by classifying it as primary or secondary. (See *Identifying primary lesions*.) A primary lesion is the initial lesion that develops. Changes in a primary lesion constitute a secondary lesion. Examples of secondary lesions include fissures, scales, crusts, scars, and excoriations.

Is it solid or fluid-filled?

Determine if the lesion is solid or fluid-filled. Macules, papules, nodules, wheals, and hives are solid lesions. Vesicles, bullae, pustules, and cysts are fluid-filled lesions. Using a flashlight or penlight will help you determine

---

Identifying primary lesions

Are you having trouble identifying your patient's lesion? Here's a quick look at three common lesions. Remember to keep a centimeter ruler handy to accurately measure the size of the lesion.

Macule
A flat circumscribed area of altered skin color, generally less than ⅜" (1 cm). Examples: freckle, flat nevus

Papule
Raised, circumscribed, solid area; generally less than ⅜". Examples: elevated nevus, wart

Vesicle
Circumscribed, elevated lesion; contains serous fluid; less than ⅜". Example: early chickenpox

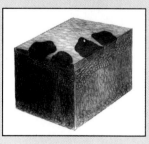
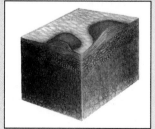
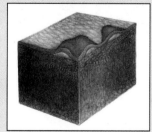

whether a lesion is solid or fluid-filled. (See *Illuminating lesions.*)

Does the fungus fluoresce?

To identify lesions that fluoresce, use a Wood's lamp, which gives out specially filtered ultraviolet light. Darken the room and then shine the light on the lesion. If the lesion looks bluish green, the patient has a fungal infection.

Learning to look at a lesion

Once you have identified the type of lesion, you'll need to describe its characteristics, pattern, location, and distribution. A detailed description will help you determine whether the lesion is a normal or pathologic skin change.

Asymmetry and borders

Examine the lesion to see if it looks the same on both sides. Also check the borders to see if they're regular or irregular. An asymmetrical lesion with an irregular border may indicate malignancy.

Color and configuration

Lesions occur in a variety of colors. Be alert for changes in those colors. For example, if a lesion has changed from tan or brown to multiple shades of tan, dark brown, black, or a mixture of red, white, and blue, the lesion might be malignant.

Pay close attention as well to the configuration and distribution of the lesion. (See *Recognizing common lesion configurations.*) Skin diseases often have typical configuration patterns. Identifying those patterns will help you determine the cause of the problem.

Diameter and drainage

Measure the exact diameter of the lesion using a centimeter ruler. If you estimate the diameter, you may not be able to determine subtle changes in size. An increase in the size or elevation of a mole over a period of many years is common and probably normal. Still, make sure to note moles that change size rapidly.

If you note drainage, document the type and amount. Also note if the lesion has a foul odor, which can indicate a superimposed infection.

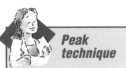

Peak technique

Illuminating lesions

Illuminating a lesion will help you see it better and learn more about its characteristics. Here are two techniques worth perfecting.

Macule or papule?
To determine whether a lesion is a macule or a papule, try this test: Reduce direct light, and shine a penlight or flashlight at a right angle to the lesion. If the light casts a shadow, the lesion is a papule. Macules are flat and won't produce a shadow.

Fluid-filled or solid?
To determine whether a lesion is fluid-filled or solid, use this technique: Place the tip of a flashlight or penlight against the side of the lesion. Fluid-filled lesions will transilluminate with a red glow. Solid lesions won't transmit light.

Recognizing common lesion configurations

Identify the configuration of your patient's skin lesion by matching it to one of these diagrams.

Discrete
Individual lesions are separate and distinct.

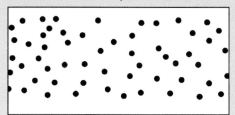

Annular
Lesions are arranged in a single ring or circle.

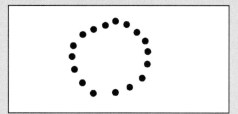

Grouped
Lesions are clustered together.

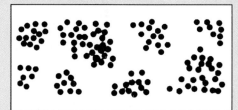

Polycyclic
Lesions are arranged in concentric circles.

Confluent
Lesions merge so that individual lesions aren't visible or palpable.

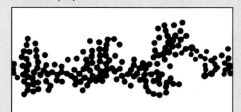

Arciform
Lesions form arcs or curves.

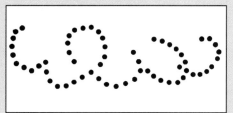

Linear
Lesions form a line.

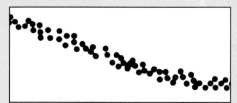

Reticular
Lesions form a meshlike network.

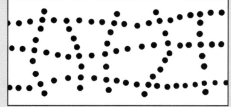

Hair

Start by inspecting and palpating the hair over the patient's entire body, not just on his head. Note the distribution, quantity, texture, and color. The quantity and distribution of head and body hair varies between patients. However, hair should be evenly distributed over the entire body.

Too much or too little?

Check for patterns of hair loss and growth. If you notice patchy hair loss, look for regrowth. Also examine the scalp for erythema, scaling, and encrustation. Excessive hair loss with scalp crusting may indicate ringworm infestation. The only way to detect scalp crusting is by using a Wood's lamp. Also note areas of excessive hair growth, which may indicate a hormone imbalance or be a sign of a systemic disorder such as Cushing's syndrome.

Having a bad hair day?

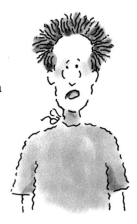

The texture of scalp hair also varies between patients. As a rule, hair should be shiny and smooth, not dry or brittle. Differences in grooming and hairstyling may affect the texture and quality of the hair. Dryness or brittleness can result from the use of harsh hair treatments or hair care products, or it might be due to a systemic illness. Extreme oiliness is usually related to an excessive production of sebum or poor grooming habits.

Nails

Assessing the nails is vital for two reasons: The appearance of nails can be a critical indicator of systemic illness, and their overall condition tells you a lot about the patient's grooming habits and ability to care for himself. Examine the nails for color, shape, thickness, consistency, and contour.

Nail that color

First, look at the color of the nails. Light-skinned people generally have pinkish nails. Dark-skinned people generally have brown nails. Brown-pigmented bands in the nail beds are normal in dark-skinned people and abnormal in light-skinned people. Yellow nails may occur in smokers as a result of nicotine stains.

Nail beds can be used to assess a patient's peripheral circulation. Press on the nail bed and then release, noting how long the color takes to return. It should return immediately, or at least within 3 seconds.

What shapely nails!

Next inspect the shape and contour of the nails. The surface of the nail bed should be either slightly curved or flat. The edges of the nail should be smooth, rounded, and clean.

The normal angle of the nail base is 160 degrees. An increase in the nail angle suggests clubbing. Curved nails are a normal variation. They may appear to be clubbed until you notice that the nail angle is still 160 degrees or less.

Finally, palpate the nail bed to check the thickness of the nail and the strength of its attachment to the bed.

Abnormal findings

Disorders of the skin, hair, and nails are classified according to cause, location, or type of lesion. Sometimes, two patients with the same diagnosis will have very different signs and symptoms, and two patients with the same signs and symptoms will have different diagnoses. Carefully document all signs and symptoms, pertinent health history, and as much information as possible from the physical examination.

Disorders of the skin

The signs and symptoms you detect during your assessment may be caused by a wide variety of skin disorders. This section describes the most common dermatoses, infestations, pigmentation disorders, skin lesions, and viral, bacterial, and fungal infections. Don't forget to refer to the chart *Evaluating skin color variations* on page 72 and the color photographs on pages 59 to 62.

Allergic disorders

These disorders result from allergic reactions and include contact dermatitis and atopic eczema.

Atopic eczema

Also known as atopic dermatitis, this form of eczema occurs in infants and adults. Generally, the patient has a family history of allergies and may have a single episode or chronic occurrences. Lesions are usually seen on the scalp, forehead, cheeks, back of the knees, and the arms, especially on the antecubital flexure.

Primary lesions include erythematous papules and vesicles that weep and ooze. Crusting may also occur. In chronic occurrences, a thickening, or lichenification, may occur in the antecubital fossa and the popliteal fossae.

Contact dermatitis

Contact dermatitis is an inflammation of the skin resulting from contact with certain irritants or allergenic substances. It can develop in any area of the body as a result of contact with soaps, deodorants, creams, shampoos, clothing, jewelry, or plants.

Primary lesions include red macules that appear as localized areas of redness, vesicles, and large, oozing bullae. Secondary lesions, such as crusting and excoriations, can result from bacterial infections.

Vascular disorders

Vascular disorders can occur in many forms, each of which produces some type of lesion. The most common vascular disorders are cherry angioma, port-wine hemangioma, purpuric lesions, telangiectases, and urticaria.

Cherry angioma

Cherry angiomas are tiny, bright red, round papules that may become brown with time. These clinically insignificant lesions occur in virtually everyone over age 30 and increase in number with age.

Port-wine hemangioma

Port-wine hemangioma, commonly called port-wine stains, are usually present at birth and often appear on the face and upper body as a flat purple mark.

Purpuric lesions

Purpuric lesions are caused by red blood cells and blood pigments in the skin, so they don't blanch under pressure.

The lesions include petechiae, ecchymoses, and hematomas.

Petechiae are red or brown pinpoint lesions often caused by capillary fragility. Diseases associated with the formation of microemboli or bleeding, such as subacute bacterial endocarditis and thrombocytopenia, can also cause petechiae.

Purpura also produces deep red or reddish purple bruising that may be caused by bleeding disorders such as disseminated intravascular coagulation.

Check out color photos on pages 59 to 62.

Telangiectases

Permanently dilated, small blood vessels, telangiectases often form a weblike pattern. For example, spider hemangiomas, a type of telangiectasis, are small, red lesions arranged in a weblike configuration. They're most commonly seen on the face, neck, and chest and may be normal or associated with pregnancy or cirrhosis.

Urticaria

Commonly known as hives, urticaria is typically acute, though you may also see the chronic form. Commonly caused by allergies, chronic and acute urticaria can also result from cancer, hyperthyroidism, and juvenile rheumatoid arthritis.

Primary lesions range from small, red papules to larger circular patterns with red borders. In severe cases, you may see vesicles and bullae. The lesions usually subside on their own, though treatment may be necessary.

Bacterial infections

The bacterial infection you'll observe most often is impetigo. A superficial infection that most often affects children, impetigo is caused by bacteria from group A beta-hemolytic streptococci or *Staphylococcus*. Primary lesions range from small vesicles to large bullae that, when ruptured, ooze a honey-colored serous fluid that can become purulent.

Crusts typically form as secondary lesions. These lesions occur most often on the face, especially near the nose and mouth, though they may also occur in the creases of the hands and elsewhere.

Fungal infections

Candidiasis and tinea infections are the most common fungal infections.

Candidiasis

Candidiasis causes lesions in the mouth, vagina, and the diaper area in infants. Candidiasis of the mouth, or thrush, appears as whitish flakes on reddened mucous membranes. You may also note fissures in the corners of the mouth.

Candidiasis of the skin, or diaper rash, occurs as scalding, red, moist patches with sharply demarcated borders and loose scales in the genital area. Candidiasis of the vagina, or vulvovaginitis, causes the same symptoms plus a milklike discharge.

Tinea infections

A group of noncandidal fungal infections, tinea infections involve the stratum corneum, nails, and hair. The lesions are usually classified according to anatomic location and can occur on:
- nonhairy parts of the body (tinea corporis)
- the groin and inner thigh (tinea cruris)
- the scalp (tinea capitis)
- the feet (tinea pedis)
- the nails (tinea unguium).

The lesions vary in appearance and may be papular, pustular, vesicular, erythematous, or scaling. They usually develop into circular or oval lesions with scaling borders.

Viral infections

The viral infections you're mostly likely to see include herpes simplex, herpes zoster, and warts.

Herpes simplex

Herpes simplex is a recurrent virus characterized by an acute, moderately painful eruption of a single group of vesicles or a fever blister. The vesicles progress to pustules and then crust. The patient may experience tingling and sensitivity around the mouth prior to eruption of the vesicles or blister.

Herpes simplex occurs in two strains: Type 1 and Type 2. If the patient has a fever blister near his mouth, he has Type 1; if the lesion appears in the genital area, he has Type 2, a sexually transmitted disease.

Herpes zoster

Herpes zoster, or shingles, is probably caused by the same virus that causes chickenpox. It appears as multiple, painful vesicles, occurring unilaterally along a cutaneous nerve, mostly on the face, neck, and thorax. The vesicles progress to pustules and then crust.

Warts

The growths known as warts or verrucae are caused by papillomavirus. The clinical diagnosis of warts varies, depending on their appearance and location.

Skin tumors

Common skin tumors include basal cell carcinoma, squamous cell carcinoma, malignant melanomas, and Kaposi's sarcoma.

Basal cell carcinoma

The most common skin cancer, basal cell carcinoma grows slowly and doesn't metastasize. It's caused by sun exposure and occurs most often on the head and neck. The most common type, noduloulcerative, produces a small, waxy-looking nodule that ulcerates, forming a central depression. Histologic studies should be done whenever basal cell carcinoma is suspected.

Squamous cell carcinoma

This malignant skin cancer is caused by direct exposure to the sun. Characterized by a raised border and a central ulcer, squamous cell carcinomas vary from fast-growing lesions to slowly developing raised growths. The degree of metastasis and malignancy also varies. This cancer can develop on any area but it's especially common on the face and neck.

Malignant melanoma

Malignant melanomas usually appear as black or purple nodules, though some are pink or red. They may have irregular or notched borders and a scaling, flaking, or oozing texture. They can develop anywhere on the body.

Some melanomas result from repeated sun exposure but more often develop in patients who have had a single, severe, blistering sunburn as children. Because most melanomas develop from preexisting nevi, always docu-

What does it all mean?

Evaluating skin color variations

To interpret your findings faster, refer to this chart.

Color	Distribution	Possible cause
Absent	• Small circumscribed areas • Generalized	• Vitiligo • Albinism
Blue	• Around lips or generalized	• Cyanosis. *Note:* In blacks, blue gingivae are normal.
Deep red	• Generalized	• Polycythemia vera (increased red blood cell count)
Pink	• Local or generalized	• Erythema (superficial capillary dilation and congestion)
Tan to brown	• Facial patches	• Chloasma of pregnancy; butterfly rash of lupus erythematosus
Tan to brown-bronze	• Generalized (not related to sun exposure)	• Addison's disease
Yellow to yellowish brown	• Sclera or generalized	• Jaundice from liver dysfunction. *Note:* In blacks, yellowish brown pigmentation of sclera is normal.
Yellow-orange	• Palms, soles, and face; not sclera	• Carotenemia (carotene in the blood)

ment changes in the size, shape, and pigment of nevi, as well as associated erythema.

Kaposi's sarcoma

This multiple hemorrhagic sarcoma usually begins on the feet and ankles. Initially, you'll notice multiple bluish red or brown nodules and plaques. Visceral lesions may develop later.

Patients infected with human immunodeficiency virus have a significantly different pattern of Kaposi's sarcoma. In those patients, the lesions are small, pink papules that usually occur on the temple or beard area but can occur anywhere. Lesions develop into raised papules or thickened, oval plaques that vary in color from red to brown. In advanced stages, violet-colored tumors cover the nose and face.

Other skin disorders

Other common skin disorders you might discover include acne, psoriasis, scabies, seborrheic keratoses, and vitiligo.

Acne

Acne is the most common skin problem in adolescence and results from oversecretion of the sebaceous glands. It usually appears on the face, chest, back, and shoulders. Primary lesions are comedones, blackheads, pustules, and cysts.

Psoriasis

The most common papulosquamous disorder you're likely to detect during your assessment is psoriasis. A chronic, recurrent disease of keratin synthesis, psoriasis commonly appears on the patient's elbows, knees, and scalp. Primary lesions consist of well-circumscribed, dry, silvery, scaling papules and plaques. About one-half of all people with psoriasis also have pitting or thickening of the skin on the elbows and knees.

Scabies

Caused by a mite that burrows under the skin, scabies commonly occurs in school-age children. It causes extreme itching and is characterized by vesicles and excoriation over the burrow sites. The most common areas for infestation are the finger webs, flexor surface of the wrists, and antecubital fossae.

Seborrheic keratoses

Seborrheic keratoses are pigmented, raised, wartlike lesions that appear primarily on the face and trunk. They're common in the elderly and caused by changes in the skin due to aging. They must be distinguished from actinic keratoses, which are faint red and scaly. Seborrheic keratoses, which gradually enlarge and occur mainly on sun-exposed areas, can become malignant.

Check out color photos on pages 59 to 62.

Vitiligo

Vitiligo is the complete absence of melanin pigment and leads to patchy areas of white or light skin. It most commonly appears on the face, neck, hands, feet, body folds, and around orifices. It can occur in any patient but is usually seen in dark-skinned people.

Disorders of the hair

Often stemming from other problems, hair disorders can cause patients emotional distress. Among the most common hair abnormalities are alopecia, folliculitis, hirsutism, pediculosis, and tinea capitis.

Alopecia

Alopecia occurs more commonly and extensively in men than in women. Diffuse hair loss, while often a normal part of aging, may occur along with pyrogenic infections, chemical trauma, ingestion of certain drugs, and endocrinopathy and other disorders. Tinea capitis, trauma, and third-degree burns can cause patchy hair loss.

Folliculitis

A superficial infection of the hair follicle, folliculitis is usually caused by staphylococci. This infection can extend to the hair bulb and is characterized by multiple pustules with hair visible at the center and an erythematous base. It usually occurs on the arms, legs, face, and buttocks.

Hirsutism

Excessive hairiness in women, or hirsutism, can develop on the body and face, affecting the patient's self-image. Localized hirsutism may occur on pigmented nevi. Generalized hirsutism can result from taking certain drugs or from endocrine problems, such as Cushing's syndrome and acromegaly.

Pediculosis

Pediculosis, or lice infestation, usually occurs on the scalp but can occur anywhere that the patient has hair. Although you may not see the mites themselves, you most likely will see their eggs (nits) in the patient's hair. This disorder causes itching and scratching and affects people of all ages. It usually results from crowded living conditions or lack of cleanliness. Head lice is particularly common in children and spreads easily in schools and day care centers.

Tinea capitis

Tinea capitis—rounded, patchy hair loss on the scalp—leaves broken hairs, pustules, and scales on the skin.

Disorders of the nails

Although many nail abnormalities are harmless, some point to serious underlying problems. Common nail problems include Beau's lines, clubbing, koilonychia, onycholysis, paronychia, and Terry's nails.

Beau's lines

Beau's lines are transverse depressions in the nail that extend to the nail bed. They occur with acute illness, malnutrition, anemia, and trauma that temporarily impairs nail function. A dent appears first at the cuticle and then moves forward as the nail grows.

Clubbing

With clubbed fingers, the proximal edge of the nail elevates so the angle is greater than 180 degrees. (See *Evaluating clubbed fingers,* page 76.) The nail will also be thickened and curved at the end, and the distal phalanx will look rounder and wider than normal. To check for clubbing, view the index finger in profile and note the angle of the nail base.

Koilonychia

Koilonychia refers to thin, spoon-shaped nails with lateral edges that tilt upward, forming a concave profile. The nails are white and opaque. This condition is associated with hypochromic anemia, chronic infections, Raynaud's disease, and malnutrition.

Onycholysis

Onycholysis is the loosening of the nail plate with separation from the nail bed, which begins at the distal groove. It's associated with minor trauma to long fingernails and disease processes, such as psoriasis, contact dermatitis, hyperthyroidism, and *Pseudomonas* infections.

What does it all mean?

Evaluating clubbed fingers

Think hypoxia when you see a patient whose fingers are clubbed. To quickly examine a patient's fingers for early clubbing, gently palpate the bases of his nails. Normally, they'll feel firm, but in early clubbing, they'll feel springy.

To evaluate late clubbing, have the patient place the first phalanges of the forefingers together, as shown. Normal nail bases are concave and create a small, diamond-shaped space when the first phalanges are opposed, as shown above.

Late clubbing
In late clubbing, however, the now convex nail bases can touch without leaving a space, as shown below. This condition is associated with pulmonary and cardiovascular disease. So when you spot clubbed fingers, think about the possible causes, such as emphysema, chronic bronchitis, lung cancer, and congestive heart failure.

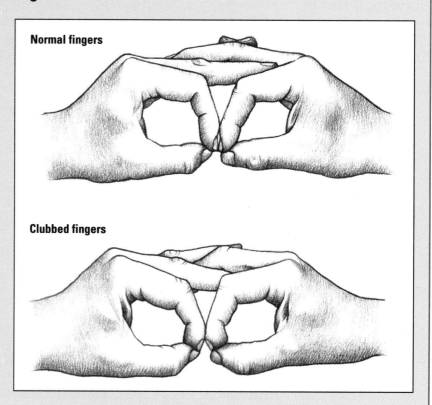

Paronychia

Causing red, swollen, tender inflammation of the nail folds, acute paronychia is usually caused by a bacterial infection. Chronic paronychia is usually caused by a fungal infection that results from a break in the cuticle and is an occupational hazard of people whose jobs involve frequently submerging their hands in water.

Terry's nails

Terry's nails are characterized by transverse bands of white that cover the nail except for a narrow zone at the distal end. Terry's nails are associated with hypoalbuminemia.

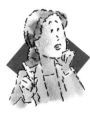

Quick quiz

1. If your patient has a skin rash, you would ask specific questions to determine whether either of the patient's parents has a history of:
- A. allergies.
- B. emphysema.
- C. Kaposi's sarcoma.

Answer: A. A family history of allergic disorders might predispose the patient to allergies, including skin rashes.

2. A Wood's lamp is used to identify:
- A. folliculitis.
- B. skin exudates.
- C. ringworm infestation.

Answer: C. A Wood's lamp is used to identify lesions that fluoresce and is the only way to identify ringworm infestation.

3. Asymmetric borders on a lesion suggest a:
- A. benign lesion.
- B. malignant lesion.
- C. probably normal variation.

Answer: B. Asymmetric borders are significant and often signal malignancy.

4. Skin temperature is best assessed with the:
- A. fingertips.
- B. back of the hand.
- C: palm of the hand.

Answer: B. The dorsal surface of the hand is the most sensitive to temperature changes.

5. A dark band is a normal finding on the nails of:
- A. elderly people.
- B. pregnant women.
- C. dark-skinned people.

Answer: C. Dark bands are normal in dark-skinned people and abnormal in light-skinned people.

6. Raised, pigmented, wartlike lesions that appear primarily on the face and trunk suggest:
- A. eczema.
- B. folliculitis.
- C. seborrheic keratoses.

Answer: C. These kinds of lesions suggest seborrheic keratoses, which gradually enlarge and occur mainly on sun-exposed areas. These lesions can become malignant.

Scoring

☆☆☆ If you answered all six items correctly, great Scot! Treat yourself to a haircut, a massage, and a movie!

☆☆ If you answered four or five items correctly, jumpin' Jupiter! Let your hair down and dance the night away!

☆ If you answered fewer than four items correctly, goodness gracious! Take a refreshing bubble bath with a hair-raising novel and a cup of java!

5

Eyes

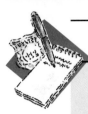

Just the facts

This chapter describes how to perform a complete eye assessment. In this chapter, you'll learn:

♦ why assessing the eyes is important

♦ about structures that make up the eye and their functions

♦ how to obtain health history information about the eyes

♦ how to perform a physical assessment of the eyes

♦ how to recognize normal and abnormal variations in the eyes.

A look at the eyes

About 70% of all sensory information reaches the brain through the eyes. Disorders in vision can interfere with a patient's ability to function independently, perceive the world, and enjoy beauty.

A thorough assessment of your patient's eyes and vision can help you identify vision problems that can affect the patient's health and quality of life. In many cases, early detection can lead to successful, sight-saving treatment.

Losing sight

Fewer people lose their sight from infections or injuries today than in the past. Still, the overall incidence of blindness is rising as the population ages. Primary causes of vision loss include diabetic retinopathy, glaucoma, cataracts, and macular degeneration — conditions more common in elderly patients than younger ones.

Younger people can lose their sight due to opportunistic infections associated with human immunodeficiency virus (HIV) and acquired immunodeficiency syndrome. The opportunistic infections toxoplasmosis and cytomegalovirus retinitis often cause blindness. Other vision disorders that may limit a person's ability to function include strabismus, amblyopia, and refractory errors.

Eye structures

The eyes are delicate sensory organs equipped with many protective structures. (See *A close look at the eye*.) On the outside, the bony orbits protect the eye from trauma. Eye-

A close look at the eye

This cross section details important anatomic structures of the eye.

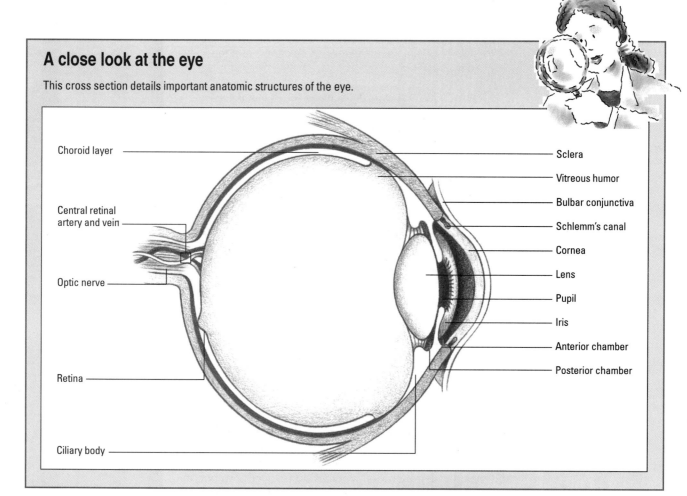

Choroid layer

Central retinal artery and vein

Optic nerve

Retina

Ciliary body

Sclera

Vitreous humor

Bulbar conjunctiva

Schlemm's canal

Cornea

Lens

Pupil

Iris

Anterior chamber

Posterior chamber

lids (or palpebrae), lashes, and the lacrimal apparatus protect the eyes from injury, dust, and foreign bodies.

Sclera, choroid, and vitreous humor

The white coating on the outside of the eyeball, the sclera, maintains the eye's size and shape. The choroid, which lines the recessed portion of the eyeball beneath the sclera, contains small arteries and veins that maintain blood supply to the eye. The vitreous humor is a thick, gelatinous material that fills the space directly behind the lens and maintains the retina's placement and the eyeball's spherical shape.

Bulbar conjunctiva and cornea

A thin, transparent membrane, the bulbar conjunctiva lines the eyelids and covers and protects the anterior portion of the eyeball. The cornea is a smooth, avascular, transparent tissue that merges with the conjunctiva at the limbus. It refracts, or bends, light rays entering the eye.

The cornea replaces the sclera over the pupil and iris and is fed by the ophthalmic branch of cranial nerve V (the trigeminal nerve). Stimulation of this nerve initiates a protective blink, the corneal reflex.

Iris

The iris is a circular, contractile disk that contains smooth and radial muscles and is perforated in the center by the pupil. Its surface consists of numerous smooth-muscle fibers of varying color. Its posterior portion contains involuntary muscles that control pupil size and regulate the amount of light entering the eye.

Lens

Located directly behind the iris at the pupillary opening, the lens consists of transparent fibers in an elastic membrane called the lens capsule. The lens refracts and focuses light onto the retina and contains no blood vessels, nerves, or connective tissue.

Pupil

The iris's central opening, the pupil is normally round and equal in size to the opposite pupil. The pupil permits light to enter the eyes. Depending on the patient's age, pupil diameter can range from ⅛" to ¼" (0.3 to 0.5 cm). Small and unresponsive to light at birth, the pupil enlarges during childhood and then progressively decreases in size throughout adulthood.

Anterior and posterior chambers

The anterior chamber is filled with a clear, watery fluid called aqueous humor. The amount of fluid in the chamber varies in an effort to maintain pressure in the eye. The pressure keeps the retina smooth to provide clear visual images. Fluid drains from the anterior chamber through Schlemm's canal.

The posterior chamber is also filled with aqueous humor and is located directly behind the iris, anterior to the lens. Like the anterior chamber, the posterior chamber helps to circulate aqueous humor and maintain pressure within the eye.

Vitreous chamber and ciliary body

The vitreous chamber, located behind the lens, occupies four-fifths of the eyeball. This chamber is filled with vitreous humor, a gelatinous substance that helps to shape the eyeball and enables it to resist extraocular pressure.

The ciliary body is the thickened part of the eye's vascular coat and joins the iris and choroid. It controls lens thickness and, with the coordinated action of the iris's muscles, regulates light passing through the lens to the retina.

Retina

The innermost region of eyeball, the retina receives visual stimuli and transmits images to the brain for processing. Four sets of retinal blood vessels—the superonasal, inferonasal, superotemporal, and inferotemporal—are visible through an ophthalmoscope.

Each set of vessels contains a transparent arteriole and vein. As these vessels leave the optic disk, they become progressively thinner, intertwining as they extend to the periphery of the retina.

Optic disk and physiologic cup

A well-defined, round or oval area measuring less than ⅛″ (0.2 cm) within the retina's nasal portion, the optic disk is the opening through which the optic nerve enters the retina. This area is called the blind spot because no light-sensitive cells are located there.

The physiologic cup is a light-colored depression within the temporal side of the optic disk where blood vessels enter the retina. It covers one-fourth to one-third of the disk but doesn't extend completely to the margin.

Photoreceptor neurons

Photoreceptor neurons make up the retina's visual receptors. Not visible through the ophthalmoscope, these receptors — some shaped like rods and some like cones — are responsible for color vision. Rods respond to low-intensity light and shades of gray. Cones respond to bright light and color.

Macula and fovea centralis

Located laterally from the optic disk, the macula is slightly darker than the rest of the retina and contains no visible retinal vessels. Because its borders are poorly defined, the macula is difficult to see on an ophthalmologic examination.

The fovea centralis, a slight depression in the retina, appears as a bright reflection when examined with an ophthalmoscope. Because the fovea contains the heaviest concentration of cones, it acts as the eye's main vision and color receptor.

Extraocular muscles

Six extraocular muscles fed by the cranial nerves control movement of the eyes. The coordinated actions of those muscles allow the eyes to move in tandem, ensuring clear vision.

Memory jogger

To remember the function and color distinction of rods and cones, picture a gray **rod** of steel (rods respond to shades of gray) or a brightly colored ice cream **cone** (cones respond to color).

Obtaining a health history

Now that you're familiar with the normal anatomy and physiology of the eye, you're ready to obtain a health history of the eyes. The most common eye-related complaints are double vision (diplopia), visual floaters, iridescent vision, vision loss, and eye pain. (See *Common eye complaints,* page 84.)

Other complaints include decreased visual acuity or clarity, defects in color vision, and difficulty seeing at night. Even if a patient's chief complaint or previous diagnosis isn't eye-related, you'll need to question him about

Common eye complaints

If your patient is seeking medical attention for a vision problem, his chief complaint will probably be one of the following disorders.

Color vision defects

The inability to see certain objects in color may indicate a problem with the rods and cones of the eye. Other causes include diseases of the optic nerve, fovea centralis, and macular area.

Decreased visual acuity

Lack of visual acuity — the ability to see clearly — is often associated with refractive errors. In nearsightedness, or myopia, the eye focuses the visual image in front of the retina, causing objects in close view to be seen clearly and those at a distance to be blurry. In farsightedness, or hyperopia, the eye focuses the visual image behind the retina, causing objects in close view to be blurry and those at a distance to be clear. Both of these problems are caused by an alteration in the shape of the eyeball.

Diplopia

Also called double vision, diplopia is caused by extraocular muscle weakness. It occurs when the visual axes aren't directed at the object of sight at the same time.

Eye pain

A complaint of eye pain needs immediate attention because it may signal an emergency. Be sure to ask the patient about the quality, duration, frequency, and onset of the pain; what causes it (for example, bright light); whether headaches accompany it; and what he does to relieve it.

Diseases that can cause eye pain include cataracts, glaucoma, foreign objects on the cornea or retina, abrasions, conjunctivitis, and refractive errors — the inability to focus light on the retina.

Iridescent vision

Iridescent vision causes the patient to see halos and rainbows in or around bright lights when he's not squinting. It can be caused by corneal edema; by a rapid increase in intraocular pressure, as with glaucoma; or by corneal abrasions, cataracts, or prolonged use of hard contact lenses.

Night blindness

The patient may complain of poor vision while driving at night, especially after bright light shines in his eyes. Night blindness, or the inability to adapt to dim light or darkness, is caused by retinal degeneration, optic nerve disease, glaucoma, or vitamin A deficiency related to malnutrition or cirrhosis.

Vision loss

Your patient may complain of central or peripheral vision loss, or he may report a scotoma — a blind spot in the visual field that's surrounded by an area of normal or decreased vision. Most vision loss results from lesions of the optic nerve, retina, or optic chiasm. The degree and location of blindness depends on the disease causing the problem or the location of the lesion. The major causes of blindness in the United States are glaucoma, untreated cataracts, retinal disease, and macular degeneration.

Visual floaters

Visual floaters are specks of varying shape and size that float through the visual field and disappear when the patient tries to look at them. They're caused by small amounts of hyaloid in the vitreous humor. Visual floaters require further investigation because they may indicate vitreous hemorrhage and retinal separation. A large, black floater that appears suddenly may indicate vitreous detachment.

his eyes and vision. *Keep in mind that poor vision can affect the patient's ability to comply with treatment.*

Asking about eyesight

To obtain an accurate history of the eyes, ask the patient first about his vision. How does he rate it? Does he wear corrective lenses? Is he having such problems as blurred vision, blind spots, floaters, double vision, pain, discharge, unusual sensitivity to light, or trouble seeing at night? Has he ever had strabismus, retinal detachment, amblyopia, eye injury, or eye surgery? Does he have allergies? When was his last eye examination?

Asking about diseases

Ask the patient if he has a history of hypertension, diabetes, cerebrovascular accident, multiple sclerosis, syphilis, or HIV. Find out if anyone in his family has glaucoma, cataracts, vision loss, or retinitis. Because a family history may predispose the patient to these conditions, he'll need frequent testing.

Asking about medications

Ask the patient what medications he takes. Some drugs can affect vision. For example, digoxin (Lanoxin) can cause a patient to see yellow halos around bright lights. Remember to ask about over-the-counter drugs, eyedrops, and eyewashes, too.

Asking about work

Ask the patient what kind of work he does and what he does for recreation. Is he exposed to chemicals, fumes, flying debris, or infectious agents? If so, does he wear eye protection? Caution all patients to wear protective eyewear when working with substances that may injure the eye.

Asking about smoking

If your patient smokes, warn him that smoking increases the risk of vascular disease, which can lead to blindness and vision damage.

Special questions for special patients

If your patient is visually impaired, ask him how well he can manage activities of daily living. Assess whether he and his family need assistance in learning to use adaptive devices or a referral to an agency that helps visually impaired people.

If your patient is a young child, your interview will vary slightly because you'll be asking the parents questions. As a result, you may receive only objective answers, not subjective responses. (See *Seeing things differently,* page 86.)

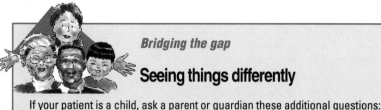

If your patient is elderly, you'll need to ask additional questions about his ability to perform daily tasks. His answers will help to guide your care.

Assessing the eyes

A complete eye assessment involves inspecting and palpating extraocular structures, testing visual acuity, assessing eye muscle function, and examining intraocular structures with an ophthalmoscope.

Before starting your examination, gather the necessary equipment, including a good light source, one or two opaque cards, an ophthalmoscope, vision-test cards, gloves, tissues, and cotton-tipped applicators. Be sure the patient is seated comfortably and that you're seated at eye level with him.

Inspecting and palpating the eyes

Start your assessment by observing the patient's face. With the scalp line as the starting point, check that his eyes are in a normal position. They should be about one-third of the way down the face and about one eye's width apart from each other. Next assess the conjunctiva, cornea, anterior chamber, iris, pupil, and eyelid.

Eyelids

Each upper eyelid should cover the top quarter of the iris so the eyes look alike. Check for an excessive amount of sclera, known as lower lid lag. Also note excessive drooping of the upper lid, known as ptosis. Ask the patient to open and close his eyes to see if they close completely. Assess the lids for redness, edema, inflammation, or lesions. Check for a stye, or hordeolum, a common eyelid lesion.

Crying or drying?

Also inspect the eyes for excessive tearing or dryness. The eyelid margins should be pink, and the eyelashes should turn upward. Observe whether the lower eyelids turn inward toward the eyeball, called entropion, or outward, called ectropion. Ask the patient to close his eyes, and then watch for fasciculation, or eyelid tremors, which may indicate hypothyroidism.

Putting a lid on it

Before palpating the eyes, explain the procedure to the patient. Then put on examination gloves. With the patient's eyes closed, gently palpate the eyelids, noting tenderness or swelling.

Examine the eyelids for lumps. Palpate the eyeball; it should feel firm, but not hard or rigid. If the eyeball feels resistant, the patient may have hyperthyroidism or a tumor. Protrusion of the eyeball, called exophthalmos or proptosis, is common in hyperthyroidism.

Next palpate the lacrimal sac by pressing your index finger against the patient's lower orbital rim near his nose. As you're pressing, look for purulent discharge or excessive tears, which could indicate blockage of the nasolacrimal duct.

Conjunctiva

Next, have your patient look up. Gently pull the lower eyelid down to inspect the bulbar conjunctiva (the delicate membrane that covers the exposed surface of the sclera). It should be clear and shiny. Note excessive redness or exudate. The bulbar conjunctiva in patients with a history of allergies may have a cobblestone appearance.

Getting an eye lift

To examine the palpebral conjunctiva (the membrane that lines the eyelids), have the patient look down. Then lift the upper lid, holding the upper lashes against the eyebrow with your finger. The palpebral conjunctiva should be uniformly pink in White patients, red-orange in Black patients, and yellow-orange in Asian patients.

With the lid still secured, inspect for color changes, foreign bodies, and edema. Also observe the sclera's color, which should be white to buff. In Black patients, you may see flecks of tan. A bluish discoloration may indicate scleral thinning.

Cornea

Then examine the cornea, shining a penlight first from both sides and then from straight ahead. The cornea should be clear and without lesions. Test corneal sensitivity by lightly touching the cornea with a wisp of cotton. (See *Tips for assessing corneal sensitivity*.)

Anterior chamber and iris

The anterior chamber of the eye is bordered anteriorly by the cornea and posteriorly by the iris. The iris should appear flat, and the cornea should appear convex. Excess pressure in the eye such as that caused by acute angle-closure glaucoma may push the iris forward, making the anterior chamber appear very small. The irises should be the same size, color, and shape.

Peak technique

Tips for assessing corneal sensitivity

To test corneal sensitivity, touch a wisp of cotton from a cotton ball to the cornea, as shown.

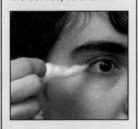

The patient should blink. If he doesn't, he may have suffered damage to the sensory fibers of cranial nerve V or to the motor fibers controlled by cranial nerve VI.

Keep in mind that people who wear contact lenses may have reduced sensitivity because they're accustomed to having foreign objects in their eyes.

Just a wisp
Remember that a wisp of cotton is the only safe object to use for this test. Even though a 4″ × 4″ gauze pad or tissue is soft, it can cause corneal abrasions and irritation.

Pupils

The pupils should be equal in size, round, and about one-quarter the size of the irises in normal room light. About one person in four has asymmetrical pupils without disease. Unequal pupils generally indicate neurologic damage, iritis, glaucoma, or the effect of certain drugs. A fixed pupil doesn't react to light and is an ominous neurologic sign.

Directly consenting pupils

Test the pupils for direct and consensual response. In a slightly darkened room, hold a penlight about 20″ (51 cm) from the patient's eyes and direct the light at the eye from the side. Note the reaction of the pupil you're testing (direct response) and the opposite pupil (consensual response). They should both react the same way. Also note sluggishness or inequality in the response. Repeat the test with the other pupil.

Accommodating pupils

To test the pupils for accommodation, place your finger approximately 4″ (10 cm) from the bridge of the patient's nose. Ask the patient to look at a fixed object in the distance and then to look at your finger. His pupils should constrict when his eyes focus on your finger.

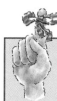

Memory jogger

To make sure that your pupil assessment is complete, think of the acronym PERRLA.

P = Pupils

E = Equal

R = Round

R = Reactive

L = Light-reacting

A = Accommodating

Testing visual acuity

To test your patient's far, near, and peripheral vision, use a Snellen chart and a near-vision chart. Before each test, ask the patient to remove corrective lenses, if he wears them.

Snellen chart

Have the patient sit or stand 20′ (6 m) from the chart, and then cover one of his eyes with an opaque object. Ask him to read the letters on one line of the chart and then to move downward to increasingly smaller lines until he can no longer discern all of the letters. Have him repeat the test with the other eye.

The Big E

Use the Snellen E chart to test visual acuity in young children and other patients who can't read. (See *Visual acuity charts,* page 90.) Cover one of the patient's eyes, point to an E on the chart, and ask the patient to point which way the letter faces. Repeat the test with the other eye.

If the patient wears corrective lenses, have him repeat the test wearing them. If the test values between the two eyes differ by two lines, such as 20/30 in one eye and 20/50 in the other, suspect an abnormality such as amblyopia, especially in children.

Near-vision chart

To test near vision, cover one of the patient's eyes with an opaque object, and hold a Rosenbaum near-vision card 14″

Visual acuity charts

The most common charts used for testing vision are the Snellen alphabet chart (left) and the Snellen E chart (right), the latter of which is used for young children and adults who can't read. Both charts are used to test distance vision and measure visual acuity. The patient reads each chart at a distance of 20' (6 m).

Recording results

Visual acuity is recorded as a fraction. The top number (20) is the distance between the patient and the chart. The bottom number is the distance from which a person with normal vision could read the line. The larger the bottom number, the poorer the patient's vision.

Age differences

In adults and children age 6 and older, normal vision is measured as 20/20. For children under age 6, normal vision varies. For children age 3 and under, normal vision is 20/50; for children age 4, 20/40; and for children age 5, 20/30.

Snellen alphabet chart

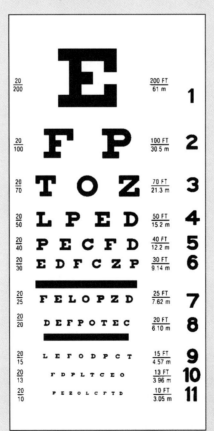

Snellen E chart

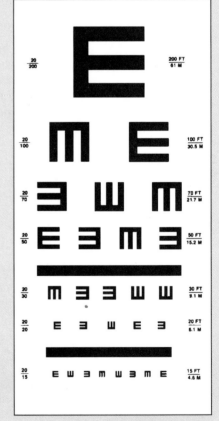

(35.6 cm) from his eyes. Have him read the line with the smallest letters he is able to distinguish. Repeat the test with the other eye. If the patient wears corrective lenses, have him repeat the test while wearing them.

Assessing eye muscle function

A thorough assessment of the eyes includes an evaluation of the extraocular muscles. To evaluate these muscles, you'll need to assess the corneal light reflex and the cardinal positions of gaze.

Corneal light reflex

To assess the corneal light reflex, ask the patient to look straight ahead; then shine a penlight on the bridge of his nose from about 12″ to 15″ (30.5 cm to 38 cm) away. The light should fall at the same spot on each cornea. If it doesn't, the eyes aren't being held in the same plane by the extraocular muscles. This finding is common in patients with lack of muscle coordination, a condition called strabismus.

Cardinal positions of gaze

Cardinal positions of gaze evaluates the oculomotor, trigeminal, and abducent nerves as well as the extraocular muscles. To perform this test, ask the patient to remain still while you hold a pencil or other small object directly in front of his nose at a distance of about 18″ (45.7 cm).

Eyeballs on the move

Ask him to follow the object with his eyes, without moving his head. Then move the object to each of the six cardinal positions, returning to the midpoint after each movement. (See *Cardinal positions of gaze*, page 92.) The patient's eyes should remain parallel as they move. Note abnormal findings such as nystagmus, the failure of one eye to follow an object.

Cover-uncover test

The third test to assess extraocular muscles is the cover-uncover test. This test usually isn't done unless you detect an abnormality during one of the two previous tests. To perform a cover-uncover test, have the patient stare at a

Cardinal positions of gaze

The diagram below shows the six cardinal positions of gaze.

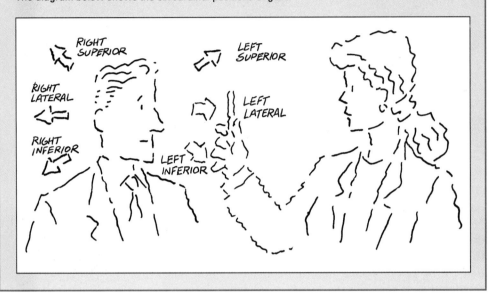

wall on the other side of the room. Then cover one eye and watch for movement in the uncovered eye. Remove the eye cover, and watch for movement again. Repeat the test with the other eye.

Eye movement while covering or uncovering the eye is considered abnormal. It may result from weak or paralyzed extraocular muscles, which may be caused by cranial nerve impairment.

Examining intraocular structures

The ophthalmoscope allows you to directly observe internal structures of the eye. To see those structures properly, you'll need to adjust the lens disk. Use the black, positive numbers on the disk to focus on near objects such as the patient's lens. Use the red, negative numbers to focus on distant objects such as the retina.

Before the examination, have the patient remove his contact lenses (unless they're clear) or eyeglasses and darken the room to dilate his pupils and make your examination easier. (See *Seeing eye to eye*.) Then ask the patient to focus on a point behind you. Tell him that you'll be moving into his visual field and blocking his view. Also explain that you'll be shining a bright light into his eye, which may be uncomfortable but isn't dangerous.

Closing in on the cornea

Set the lens disk at zero, and hold the ophthalmoscope about 12″ (30.5 cm) from the patient's eye and slightly lateral to it. Locate the red reflex, a reflection of light off the retina, which indicates a clear cornea and lens.

Now, move the ophthalmoscope closer to the lens disk. Adjust the lens disk so you can focus on the lens and anterior chamber. Look for clouding, foreign matter, or opacities. If the lens is opaque, indicating cataracts, you may not be able to complete the examination.

Rotating to the retinal structures

To examine the retina, start with the dial turned to zero. As you rotate the dial, observe the vitreous body to be sure it's transparent. The first retinal structures you'll see are the blood vessels; rotate the dial into the negative numbers to focus on them. The arteries will look thinner and brighter than the veins.

Follow one of the vessels along its path toward the nose until you reach the optic disk, where all vessels in the eye originate. Note all arteriovenous crossings, and watch for tapering of the veins, which might indicate arteriovenous nicking, a sign of hypertension.

Diggin' the disk and depression

The optic disk is a slightly concave, creamy pink to yellow-orange structure with clear borders and a round-to-oval shape. With practice, you'll be able to identify the physiologic cup, a small depression that occupies about one-third of the disk's diameter. The nasal border of the disk may be somewhat blurred.

Riveting on the retina

Then, completely scan the retina by following four blood vessels from the optic disk to different peripheral areas. (See *A close look at the retina,* page 94.) The retina should have a uniform color and be free from scars and pigmentation. As you scan, note arteriovenous crossings.

Movin' in on the macula

Finally, move the light laterally from the optic disk to locate the macula, the part of the eye most sensitive to light.

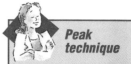

Peak technique

Seeing eye to eye

This illustration shows the correct position for the examiner and the patient when an ophthalmoscope is used to examine the internal structures of the eye.

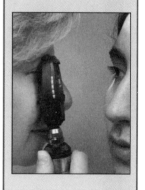

It appears as a bright spot of light, free from blood vessels. Your view may be fleeting because most patients can't tolerate having a beam of light fall on the macula. If you locate it, ask the patient to shift his gaze into the light.

Abnormal findings

Common abnormalities you may detect during an eye assessment include periorbital edema, ptosis, acute hordeolum, conjunctivitis, cataract, macular degeneration, diabetic retinopathy, glaucoma, irregular pupils, strabismus,

A close look at the retina

This illustration shows the complex anatomy of the retina and its structures.

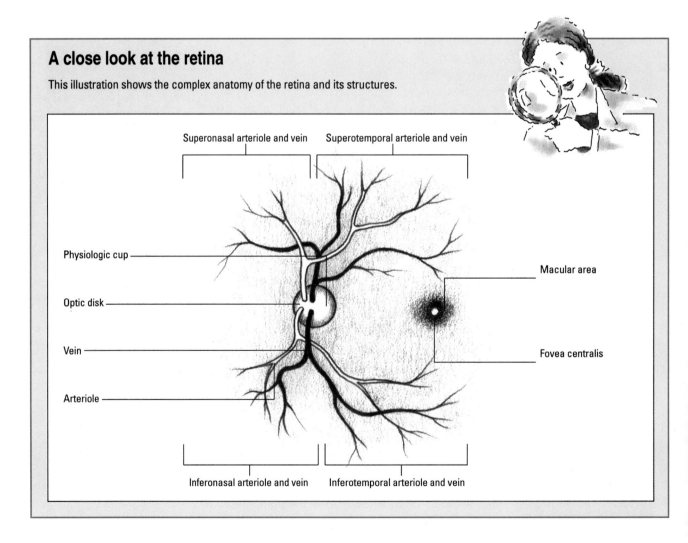

Superonasal arteriole and vein

Superotemporal arteriole and vein

Physiologic cup

Optic disk

Vein

Arteriole

Macular area

Fovea centralis

Inferonasal arteriole and vein

Inferotemporal arteriole and vein

arteriolar narrowing, and arteriovenous nicking. (See *Recognizing common eye disorders*.) Let's check them out one at a time.

Puffy periorbital edema

Swelling around the eyes, or periorbital edema, may result from allergies, local inflammation, fluid-retaining disorders, or crying.

Tired-looking ptosis

Ptosis, or a drooping upper eyelid, may be caused by an interruption in sympathetic innervation to the eyelid, muscle weakness, or damage to the oculomotor nerve.

Stye-lish acute hordeolum

Also called a stye, acute hordeolum is a bacterial infection in a sebaceous gland on the eyelid. The affected area becomes reddened and tender, and you may observe a green-yellow discharge.

Clearly visible conjunctivitis

In conjunctivitis, the blood vessels of the conjunctiva become inflamed and clearly visible to the unaided eye. The patient may complain of irritation, and you may note a discharge. A clear, watery discharge usually indicates an allergic or viral cause. A purulent discharge usually indicates a bacterial infection.

Cloudy cataract

During your examination, you may observe lens opacities, or cataracts. Cataracts are typically associated with aging.

Mixed up macular degeneration

Macular degeneration occurs in two forms: atrophic and exudative. The formation of drusen — small, raised, yellow spots in the macula — is characteristic of the atrophic form. In the exudative form, subretinal hemorrhage and fluid accumulation occur, leading to retinal scarring.

Dangerous diabetic retinopathy

This condition occurs in two forms: nonproliferative and proliferative retinopathy. In nonproliferative, or background, retinopathy, microaneurysms and small retinal hemorrhages appear in the macular area. In proliferative

---

Recognizing common eye disorders

During an eye examination, you may observe any of a number of abnormalities. These illustrations show some of those abnormal findings.

Periorbital edema

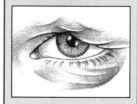

Ptosis

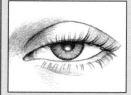

Acute hordeolum

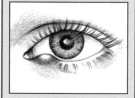

Cataract

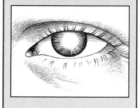

retinopathy, new blood vessels and fibrous tissue grow along the retinal surface.

Grievous glaucoma

Symptoms of chronic, open-angle glaucoma include mild aching in the eyes, loss of peripheral vision, and halos around lights. In acute angle-closure glaucoma, eye pain is unilateral, and pupils are moderately dilated and nonreactive to light. This form causes blindness in 3 to 5 days if left untreated. Early detection of glaucoma can be accomplished through tonometry. (See *Tonometry*.)

Irascible irregular pupils

A patient with glaucoma will have an irregularly shaped pupil if he has had an iridectomy, an excision of part of the iris. In addition, some people are born with a congenital abnormality in pupil shape, a condition called dyscoria.

Flimsy strabismus

In strabismus, the eyes deviate from their normal gazing position. This condition may result from extraocular muscle weakness or paralysis or from an imbalance in ocular tone. It's common in children, and if detected early, can be corrected without surgery.

Angular arteriolar narrowing

Typically, arterioles are between two-thirds and three-fourths the width of veins and have a brighter appearance. When these minute arteries narrow, they appear to be about one-half as wide as veins. Arteriolar narrowing is common in patients with hypertension.

Nasty arteriovenous nicking

In arteriovenous nicking, a vein appears to taper where the arteriole crosses it. This abnormality is common in patients with poorly controlled hypertension.

Tonometry

An effective screen for early detection of glaucoma, tonometry also provides an indirect measurement of intraocular pressure. A rise in intraocular pressure may cause the eyeball to harden and become more resistant to extraocular pressure.

Types of tonometry

Indentation tonometry tests this resistance by measuring how deeply a known weight depresses the cornea. Applanation tonometry provides the same information by measuring the amount of force required to flatten a known area of the cornea.

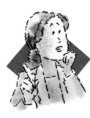

Quick quiz

1. The normal reaction to a corneal sensitivity test is:
A. blinking.
B. coughing.
C. pupil dilation.

Answer: A. The normal response to a corneal sensitivity test is blinking. Remember that a wisp of cotton is the only material safe enough to use for this test.

2. Besides trauma, unequal pupils can be the result of:
A. a cataract.
B. an iridectomy.
C. severe conjunctivitis.

Answer: B. When part of the iris is excised, an iridectomy, the result is an irregular pupil. Unequal pupils are also normal in some people.

3. Cone receptors are mainly responsible for sensing:
A. light.
B. color.
C. shapes.

Answer: B. Cones aid in color recognition and are located in the fovea centralis.

4. To determine a patient's visual acuity, you would use the:
A. Snellen chart.
B. cover-uncover test.
C. corneal light reflex test.

Answer: A. The Snellen chart tests visual acuity by having the patient read a series of letters. The Snellen E chart contains only the letter *E* and can be used for children and patients who don't read.

5. The red reflex seen during an ophthalmoscope examination is the result of:
A. an increase in intraocular pressure.
B. incorrect adjustment of the diopter.
C. light from the scope hitting the retina.

Answer: C. The red reflex results from light reflecting off the retina. To test for the reflex, shine the ophthalmoscope light at the patient's pupil from a distance of about 12″ (30.5 cm) and at a slight angle.

6. Compared with the size of a child's pupils, the size of an adult's pupils is:

    A. smaller.

    B. larger.

    C. the same throughout life.

Answer: A. Pupils are small and unresponsive to light at birth. They enlarge during childhood and progressively decrease in size throughout adulthood and into old age.

Scoring

✫✫✫   If you answered all six items correctly, terrific! You're a star pupil!

✫✫   If you answered four or five items correctly, super! You've really got vision!

✫   If you answered fewer than four items correctly, that's OK! To us, you're truly a sight for sore eyes! (We just couldn't resist!)

6

Ears, nose, and throat

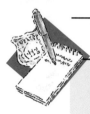

Just the facts

This chapter describes how to do a complete assessment of the ears, nose, and throat. In this chapter, you'll learn:

♦ about the structures that make up the ear, nose, and throat and their functions

♦ how to obtain an ear, nose, and throat health history from your patient

♦ how to perform an assessment of the ear, nose, and throat

♦ how to recognize ear, nose, and throat abnormalities and what causes them.

A look at the ears, nose, and throat

The three senses — hearing, smell, and taste — allow us to communicate with others, connect with the world around us, and take pleasure in life. Because these senses play such vital roles in daily life, you'll need to thoroughly assess a patient's ears, nose, and throat.

Besides revealing impairments in hearing, smell, and taste, your assessment also can uncover important clues to physical problems in the patient's integumentary, musculoskeletal, cardiovascular, respiratory, immune, and neurologic systems.

To perform an accurate physical assessment, you'll need to understand the anatomy and physiology of the ears, nose, and throat. Let's take them one by one.

Ears

The ear is divided into three parts: external, middle, and inner. (See *A close look at the ear*.) The anatomy and physiology of each part play separate but important roles in hearing.

A close look at the ear

Use this illustration to review the structures of the ear.

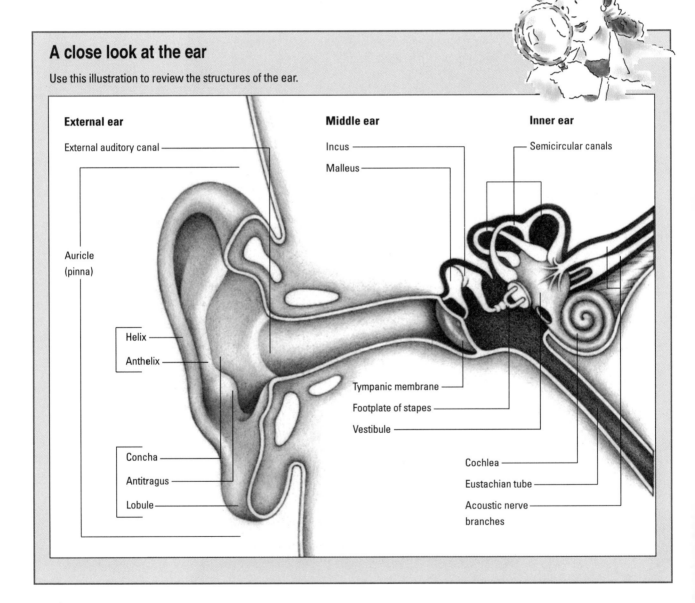

External ear

External auditory canal

Auricle (pinna)

Helix

Anthelix

Concha

Antitragus

Lobule

Middle ear

Incus

Malleus

Tympanic membrane

Footplate of stapes

Vestibule

Inner ear

Semicircular canals

Cochlea

Eustachian tube

Acoustic nerve branches

External ear

The flexible external ear consists mainly of elastic carti-lage. This part of the ear contains the ear flap, also known as the auricle or pinna, and the auditory canal. The outer third of this canal has a bony framework.

Middle ear

The tympanic membrane separates the external and mid-dle ear. This pearl gray structure consists of three layers: fibrous tissue, skin, and a mucous membrane. Its upper portion, the pars flaccida, has little support; its lower por-tion, the pars tensa, is held taut. The center, or umbo, is at-tached to the tip of the long process of the malleus on the other side of the tympanic membrane.

A small, air-filled structure, the middle ear performs three vital functions:
• It transmits sound vibrations across the bony ossicle chain to the inner ear.
• It protects the auditory apparatus from intense vibra-tions.
• It equalizes the air pressure on both sides of the tym-panic membrane to prevent it from rupturing.

Those bones, those bones, those wee small bones

The middle ear contains three small bones of the auditory ossicles: the malleus, or hammer; the incus, or anvil; and the stapes, or stirrup. These bones are linked like a chain and vibrate in place. The long process of the malleus fits into the incus, forming a true joint, and allows the two structures to move as a single unit. The proximal end of the stapes fits into the oval window, an opening that joins the middle and inner ear.

A tube with connections

The eustachian tube connects the middle ear with the na-sopharynx, equalizing air pressure on either side of the tympanic membrane. This tube also connects the ear's sterile area to the nasopharynx.

A normally functioning eustachian tube keeps the middle ear free from contaminants from the nasopharynx. Upper respiratory tract infections can affect the tube by obstructing middle ear drainage and causing otitis media or effusion.

Inner ear

The inner ear consists of closed, fluid-filled spaces within the temporal bone. It contains the bony labyrinth, which includes three connected structures: the vestibule, the semicircular canals, and the cochlea. These structures are lined with the membranous labyrinth. A fluid called perilymph fills the space between the bony labyrinth and the membranous labyrinth.

The vestibule and semicircular canals help maintain equilibrium. The cochlea, a spiral chamber that resembles a snail shell, is the organ of hearing. The organ of Corti, part of the membranous labyrinth, contains hair cells that receive auditory sensations.

Here's how we hear

When sound waves reach the external ear, structures there transmit the waves through the auditory canal to the tympanic membrane, where they cause a chain reaction among the structures of the middle and inner ear. Finally, the cochlear branch of the acoustic nerve (cranial nerve VIII) transmits the vibrations to the temporal lobe of the cerebral cortex, where the brain interprets the sound.

Here's how we stay in balance

Besides controlling hearing, structures in the middle and inner ear control balance. The semicircular canals of the inner ear contain cristae — hairlike structures that respond to body movements. Endolymph fluid bathes the cristae.

When a person moves, the cristae bend, releasing impulses through the vestibular portion of the acoustic nerve to the brain, which controls balance. When a person is stationary, nerve impulses to the brain orient him to this position, and the pressure of gravity on the inner ear helps him maintain balance.

Nose

The nose is more than the sensory organ of smell. It also plays a key role in the respiratory system, by filtering, warming, and humidifying inhaled air. When you assess the nose, you'll often assess the paranasal sinuses, too.

Right under — and on — your nose

The lower two-thirds of the external nose consists of flexible cartilage, and the upper one-third is rigid bone. Posteriorly, the internal nose merges with the pharynx. Anteriorly, it merges with the external nose.

The internal and external nose are divided vertically by the nasal septum, which is straight at birth and in early life but becomes slightly deviated or deformed in almost every adult. Only the posterior end, separating the posterior nares, remains constantly in the midline.

Just nosing around

Air entering the nose passes through the vestibule, lined with coarse hair that helps filter out dust. Olfactory receptors lie above the vestibule in the roof of the nasal cavity and the upper one-third of the septum. Known as the olfactory region, this area is rich in capillaries and mucus-producing goblet cells that help warm, moisten, and clean inhaled air.

Further along the nasal passage are the superior, middle, and inferior turbinates. Separated by grooves called meatus, the curved bony turbinates and their mucosal covering ease breathing by warming, filtering, and humidifying inhaled air.

Singling out the sinuses

Four pairs of paranasal sinuses open into the internal nose, including the:
• maxillary sinuses, located on the cheeks below the eyes
• frontal sinuses, located above the eyebrows
• ethmoidal and sphenoidal sinuses, located behind the eyes and nose in the head.

You'll be able to assess the maxillary and frontal sinuses, but the ethmoidal and sphenoidal sinuses aren't readily accessible. (See *A close look at the nose and mouth,* page 104.)

The small openings between the sinuses and the nasal cavity can become obstructed easily because they're lined with mucous membranes that can become inflamed and swollen.

Throat

The throat, or pharynx, is divided into the nasopharynx, the oropharynx, and the laryngopharynx. Located within

A close look at the nose and mouth

These illustrations show the anatomic structures of the nose, mouth, and oropharynx.

Nose and mouth

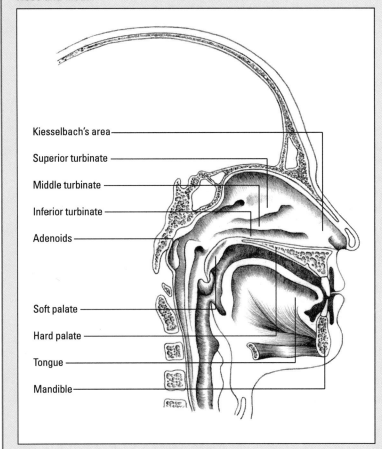

Kiesselbach's area

Superior turbinate

Middle turbinate

Inferior turbinate

Adenoids

Soft palate

Hard palate

Tongue

Mandible

Mouth and oropharynx

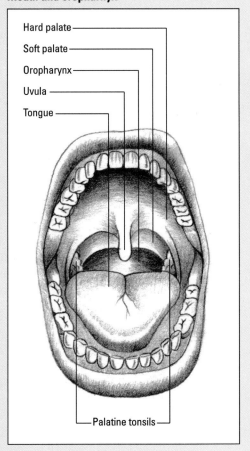

Hard palate

Soft palate

Oropharynx

Uvula

Tongue

Palatine tonsils

the throat are the hard and soft palates, the uvula, and the tonsils. The mucous membrane lining the throat normally is bright pink to light red and smooth.

Running neck and neck

The neck is formed by the cervical vertebrae and the major neck and shoulder muscles, together with their ligaments. Other important structures of the neck include the trachea, thyroid gland, and chains of lymph nodes.

The thyroid gland lies in the anterior neck, just below the larynx. Its two cone-shaped lobes are located on either side of the trachea and have a connecting isthmus below the cricoid cartilage, which gives the gland its butterfly shape. The largest endocrine gland, the thyroid produces the hormones triiodothyronine (T_3) and thyroxine (T_4), which affect the metabolic reactions of every cell in the body.

Obtaining a health history

To investigate a chief complaint about the ears, nose, or throat, ask questions about the onset, location, duration, and characteristics of the symptom as well as what aggravates and relieves it.

Asking about the ears

The most common ear complaints are hearing loss, tinnitus, pain, discharge, and dizziness. Hearing loss and tinnitus are usually caused by long-term problems. Pain, discharge, and dizziness usually result from short-term conditions.

Ask the patient if he feels dizzy or off balance, if he has had an ear problem or injury before, or if anyone in his family has ear or hearing problems. Also ask if he has been ill recently or if he has a chronic disorder. For example, diabetes can cause hearing loss, and hypertension can cause high-pitched tinnitus.

If the patient has a chronic disorder, ask about treatment and medications. Certain antibiotics and other medications can cause hearing loss.

When allergies hit

Ask the patient if he has allergies. Serous otitis media, or inflammation of the middle ear, is common in people with environmental or seasonal allergies. Otitis externa, or inflammation of the external ear, can be caused by allergic reactions to hair dyes, cosmetics, perfumes, and other personal care products.

Asking about the nose

The most common complaints about the nose include nasal stuffiness, nasal discharge, and epistaxis, or nosebleed. Ask if the patient has had any of these problems.

Also ask about frequent colds, hay fever, headaches, and sinus trouble. Ask whether certain conditions or places seem to cause or aggravate the patient's problem. Ask if he has ever had nose or head trauma.

Environmental allergies can cause nasal stuffiness and discharge, and stagnant nasal discharge can act as a culture medium and lead to sinusitis and other infections. Also ask about the color and consistency of the discharge.

Asking about the mouth, throat, and neck

Ask the patient if he has bleeding or sore gums, mouth or tongue ulcers, a bad taste in his mouth, bad breath, toothaches, loose teeth, frequent sore throats, hoarseness, or facial swelling. Also ask whether he smokes or uses other types of tobacco. If the patient is having neck problems, ask if he has neck pain or tenderness, neck swelling, or trouble moving his neck.

Related questions

After asking specific questions about the ears, nose, mouth, throat, and neck, ask questions about the patient's general health. Be alert for responses that might indicate a thyroid disorder. Hyperthyroidism can cause heat intolerance, weight loss, and a short menstrual pattern with scant flow. Hypothyroidism can cause cold intolerance, weight gain, an increase in menstrual pattern and flow and, in extreme cases, bradycardia and dyspnea from low cardiac output. Ask the patient these questions about possible signs and symptoms:
• Have you noticed changes in the way you tolerate hot and cold weather?
• Has your weight changed recently?
• Do you have breathing problems or feel as if your heart is skipping beats?
• Have you noticed a change in your menstrual pattern?

Assessing the ears, nose, and throat

Examining the ears, nose, and throat mainly involves using the techniques of inspection, palpation, and auscultation. An ear assessment also requires the use of an otoscope and hearing acuity tests.

Examining the ears

To assess your patient's ears, you'll need to inspect and palpate the external structures, perform an otoscopic examination of the ear canal, and test his hearing acuity.

External observations

Begin by observing the ears for position and symmetry. The top of the ear should line up with the outer corner of the eye, and the ears should look symmetrical, with the angle of attachment no more than 10 degrees. Both ears should be the same shape and color as the face.

Oddly shaped ears

Auricles that protrude from the head, or "lop" ears, are fairly common and don't affect hearing ability. However, low set ears commonly accompany congenital disorders, including kidney problems.

Analyzing the auricle

Inspect the auricle for lesions, drainage, nodules or redness. Pull the helix back and note if it is tender. If pulling the ear back hurts the patient, he may have otitis externa.

Then inspect and palpate the mastoid area behind each auricle, noting tenderness, redness, or warmth. Finally, inspect the opening of the ear canal, noting discharge, redness, or odor. Patients normally have varying amounts of hair and cerumen, or earwax, in the ear canal.

Otoscopic examination

Part two of your ear assessment involves examining the patient's auditory canal, tympanic membrane, and malleus with the otoscope. (See *Using an otoscope*, page 108.) Before inserting the speculum into the patient's ear canal, check the opening for foreign particles or discharge.

Then palpate the tragus — the cartilaginous projection anterior to the external opening of the ear — and pull the auricle up. If this area is tender, don't insert the speculum. The patient could have otitis externa, and inserting the speculum could be painful.

Insert speculum A into ear B

To insert the speculum of the otoscope, tilt the patient's head away from you. Then grasp the superior posterior

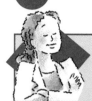

Peak technique

Using an otoscope

Here's how to use an otoscope to examine the ears.

Inserting the speculum

Before inserting the speculum into the patient's ear, straighten the ear canal by grasping the auricle and pulling it up and back, as shown.

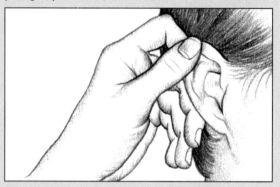

Positioning the scope

To examine the ear's external canal, hold the otoscope with the handle parallel to the patient's head, as shown. Bracing your hand firmly against his head keeps you from hitting the canal with the speculum.

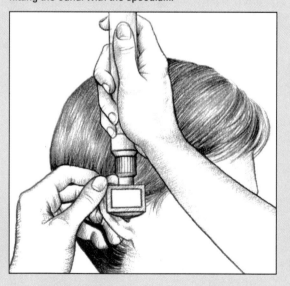

Viewing the structures

When the otoscope is positioned properly, you should see the tympanic membrane structures shown here.

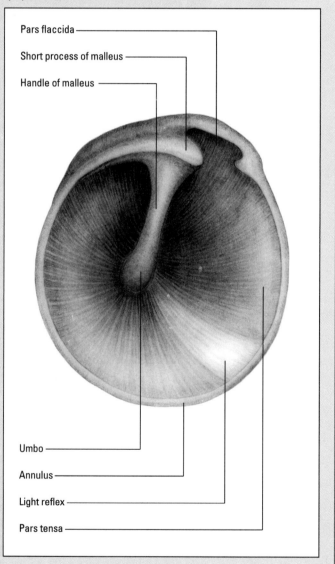

Pars flaccida

Short process of malleus

Handle of malleus

Umbo

Annulus

Light reflex

Pars tensa

auricle with your thumb and index finger and pull it up and back to straighten the canal. Because everyone's ear canal is shaped differently, vary the angle of the speculum until you can see the tympanic membrane. If your patient is a child under age 3, pull the auricle down to get a good view of the membrane.

Go gently into that good ear canal

Insert the speculum to about one-third its length when inspecting the canal. Be sure to insert it gently because the inner two-thirds of the canal is sensitive to pressure. Note the color of the cerumen. Cerumen that's grayish brown and dry-looking is old. The external canal should be free from inflammation and scaling.

If your view of the tympanic membrane is obstructed by excessive cerumen, don't try to remove it with an instrument or you could cause the patient excessive pain. Instead, use ceruminolytic drops and warm water irrigation, as ordered.

Swivel the speculum

You may need to carefully rotate the speculum for a complete view of the tympanic membrane. The membrane should be pearl gray and glistening. The annulus should be white and denser than the rest of the membrane. Inspect the membrane carefully for bulging, retraction, bleeding, lesions, or perforations, especially at the periphery.

What time is your light reflex?

Now, examine the membrane for the light reflex. The light reflex in the right ear should be between 4 and 6 o'clock; in the left ear, it should be between 6 and 8 o'clock. If the reflex is displaced or absent, the patient's tympanic membrane may be bulging, inflamed, or retracted.

Finally, look for the bony landmarks. The malleus will appear as a dense, white streak at the 12 o'clock position. At the top of the light reflex, you'll find the umbo, the inferior point of the malleus.

Hearing acuity tests

The last part of an ear assessment is testing the patient's hearing, using Weber's and Rinne's tests. These tests assess conduction hearing loss — impaired sound transmission to the inner ear — and sensorineural hearing loss — impaired auditory nerve conduction or inner ear function.

Weber's test

Weber's test uses a tuning fork to evaluate bone conduction. The tuning fork should be tuned to the frequency of normal human speech, 512 cycles/second.

To perform Weber's test, strike the tuning fork lightly against your hand, and then place the fork on the patient's forehead at the midline or on the top of his head. If he hears the tone equally well in both ears, record this as a normal Weber's test. If he hears the tone better in one ear, record the result as right or left lateralization.

During lateralization, the tone sounds louder in the ear with hearing loss because bone conducts the tone to the ear. Because the unaffected ear picks up other sounds, it doesn't hear the tone as clearly.

Rinne's test

Perform Rinne's test after Weber's test, to compare air conduction of sound with bone conduction of sound. To do this test, strike the tuning fork against your hand, and then place it over the patient's mastoid process. (See *Positioning the tuning fork*.) Ask him to tell you when the tone stops, and note this time in seconds. Next, move the still-vibrating tuning fork to the opening of the ear without touching the ear. Ask him to tell you when the tone stops. Note the time in seconds.

The patient should hear the air-conducted tone twice as long as he hears the bone-conducted tone. If he doesn't hear the air-conducted tone longer than the bone-conducted tone, he has a conductive hearing loss in the affected ear.

Examining the nose and sinuses

A complete examination of the nose also includes checking the sinuses. To perform this examination, use the techniques of inspection and palpation.

Inspecting and palpating the nose

Begin by observing the patient's nose for position, symmetry, and color. Note variations, such as discoloration, swelling, or deformity. Variations in size and shape are

Peak technique

Positioning the tuning fork

These illustrations show how to hold a tuning fork to test a patient's hearing.

Weber's test
With the tuning fork vibrating lightly, position the tip on the patient's forehead at the midline, as shown. Or place the tuning fork on the top of the patient's head.

Rinne's test
Strike the tuning fork against your hand, and then hold it behind the patient's ear, as shown. When your patient tells you the tone has stopped, move the still-vibrating tuning fork to the opening of his ear.

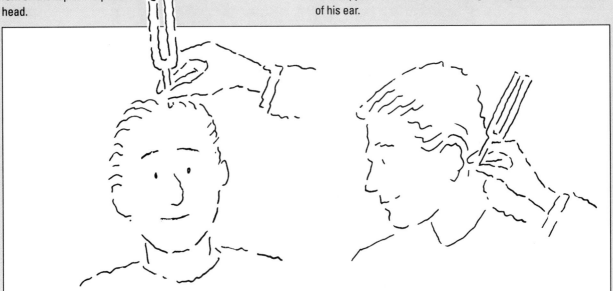

largely due to differences in cartilage and in the amount of fibroadipose tissue.

Observe for nasal discharge or flaring. If discharge is present, note the color, quantity, and consistency. If you notice flaring, observe for other signs of respiratory distress.

Hmmm, smells like ...

To test nasal patency and olfactory nerve (cranial nerve I) function, ask the patient to block one nostril and inhale a familiar aromatic substance through the other nostril. Possible substances include soap, coffee, citrus, tobacco, or

Peak technique

Inspecting the nostrils

The illustration below shows the proper placement of the nasal speculum during direct inspection and the structures you should be able to see during this examination.

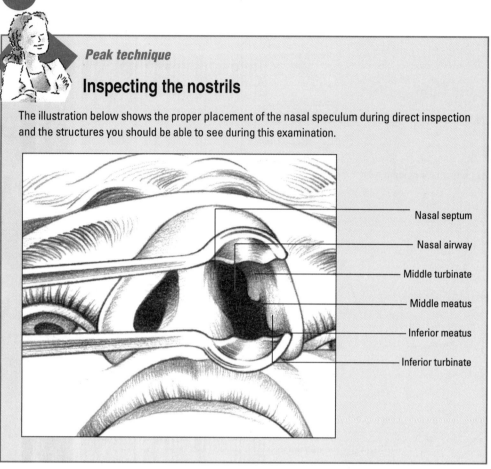

Nasal septum

Nasal airway

Middle turbinate

Middle meatus

Inferior meatus

Inferior turbinate

nutmeg. Ask him to identify the aroma. Then repeat the process with the other nostril, using a different aroma.

Turn up the patient's nose

Now, inspect the nasal cavity. Ask the patient to tilt his head back slightly, and then push the tip of his nose up. Use the light from the otoscope to illuminate his nasal cavities. Check for severe deviation or perforation of the nasal septum. Examine the vestibule and turbinates for redness, softness, and discharge.

A light at the end of the speculum

Examine the nostrils by direct inspection, using a nasal speculum and a penlight or small flashlight. Have the patient sit in front of you with his head tilted back. Put on gloves, and insert the tip of the closed nasal speculum into one nostril to the point where the blade widens. Slowly open the speculum as wide as possible without causing discomfort. Shine the flashlight in the nostril to illuminate the area.

Observe the color and patency of the nostril, and check for exudate. (See *Inspecting the nostrils*.) The mucosa should be moist, pink to light red, and free from lesions and polyps. After inspecting one nostril, close the speculum, remove it, and inspect the other nostril.

Thumb his nose

Finally, palpate the patient's nose with your thumb and forefinger, assessing for pain, tenderness, swelling, and deformity.

Examining the sinuses

Next examine the sinuses. Remember, only the frontal and maxillary sinuses are accessible; you won't be able to palpate the ethmoidal and sphenoidal sinuses. However, if the frontal and maxillary sinuses are infected, you can assume that the other sinuses are, too.

Tell me if it hurts

Begin by checking for swelling around the eyes, especially over the sinus area. Then palpate the sinuses, checking for tenderness. (See *Palpating the maxillary sinuses*.) To palpate the frontal sinuses, place your thumbs above the patient's eyes just under the bony ridges of the upper orbits and place your fingertips on his forehead. Apply gentle pressure. Next palpate the maxillary sinuses.

You can also assess maxillary sinuses by transillumination. (See *Transilluminating the sinuses*, page 114.) Transillumination can help reveal tumors and obstructions.

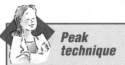

Peak technique

Palpating the maxillary sinuses

To palpate the maxillary sinuses, gently press your thumbs on each side of the nose just below the cheekbones, as shown. The illustration also shows the location of the frontal sinuses.

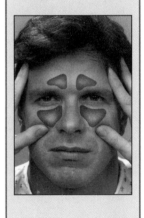

Examining the mouth, throat, and neck

Assessing the mouth and throat requires the techniques of inspection and palpation. Assessing the neck also involves auscultation.

Advice from the experts

Transilluminating the sinuses

Transillumination of the sinuses helps detect sinus tumors and obstruction and requires only a penlight. Before you start, darken the room and have the patient close his eyes.

Frontal sinuses
Place the penlight on the supraorbital ring, and direct the light upward to illuminate the frontal sinuses just above the eyebrow, as shown.

Maxillary sinuses
Place the penlight on the patient's cheekbone just below his eye, and ask him to open his mouth. The light should transilluminate easily and equally.

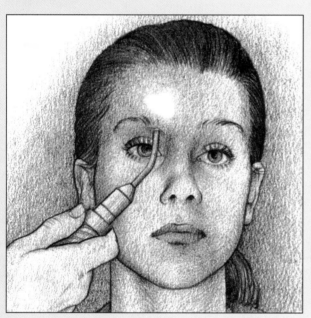

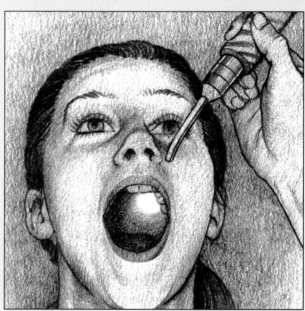

Assessing the mouth and throat

First, inspect the patient's lips. They should be pink, moist, symmetrical, and without lesions. Put on gloves and palpate the lips for lumps or surface abnormalities.

Use a tongue blade and a bright light to inspect the oral mucosa. Have the patient open his mouth, and then place the tongue blade on top of his tongue. The oral mucosa should be pink, smooth, moist, and free from lesions and unusual odors.

Next observe the gingivae, or gums: They should be pink, moist, have clearly defined margins at each tooth, and not be retracted. Inspect the teeth, noting their number, condition, and whether any are missing or crowded.

Give the tongue the once-over

Finally, inspect the tongue. It should be midline, moist, pink, and free from lesions. The posterior surface should be smooth, and the anterior surface should be slightly rough with small fissures. The tongue should move easily in all directions, and it should lie straight to the front at rest.

Ask the patient to raise the tip of his tongue and touch his palate directly behind his front teeth. Inspect the ventral surface of the tongue and the floor of the mouth. Next, wrap a piece of gauze around the tip of the tongue and move the tongue first to one side then the other to inspect the lateral borders. They should be smooth and even-textured.

Say "Ahhhh"

Inspect the patient's oropharynx by asking him to open his mouth while you shine the penlight on the uvula and palate. You may need to insert a tongue blade into the mouth and depress the tongue. The uvula and oropharynx should be pink and moist, without inflammation or exudates. The tonsils should be pink and nonhypertrophied. Ask the patient to say "ah," and then observe for movement of the soft palate and uvula.

Check the gag

Finally, palpate the lips, tongue, and oropharynx. Note lumps, lesions, ulcers, or edema of the lips or tongue. Assess the patient's gag reflex by gently touching the back of the pharynx with a cotton-tipped applicator or the tongue blade. This should produce a bilateral response.

Inspecting and palpating the neck

First, observe the patient's neck. It should be symmetrical and the skin should be intact. No visible pulsations, masses, swelling, venous distention, or thyroid or lymph node enlargement should be present. Ask the patient to move his neck through the entire range of motion and to shrug his shoulders. Also ask him to swallow. Note rising of the larynx, trachea, or thyroid.

Palpate the lymph nodes

Palpate the patient's neck to gather further data. Using the finger pads of both hands, bilaterally palpate the chain of lymph nodes under the patient's chin in the preauricular area; then proceed to the area under and behind the ears. (See *Locating lymph nodes*.) Assess the nodes for size, shape, mobility, consistency, and tenderness, comparing nodes on one side with those on the other.

Palpate the carotid artery

Next gently palpate the carotid artery to check the patient's pulse rate and blood flow. *Remember: Check the*

Peak technique

Locating lymph nodes

This illustration shows the location of lymph nodes in the patient's head and neck.

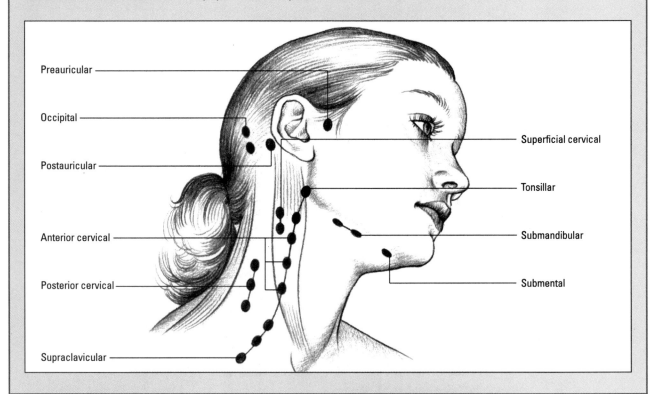

carotid arteries one side at time. Palpating both at once can trigger severe bradycardia.

Palpate the trachea

Then palpate the trachea, normally located midline in the neck. Place your thumbs along each side of the trachea near the lower part of the neck. Assess whether the distance between the trachea's outer edge and the sternocleidomastoid muscle is equal on both sides.

Palpate the thyroid

To palpate the thyroid, stand behind the patient and put your hands around his neck, with the fingers of both hands over the lower trachea. Ask him to swallow as you feel the thyroid isthmus. The isthmus should rise with swallowing because it lies across the trachea, just below the cricoid cartilage.

Displace the thyroid to the right and then to the left, palpating both lobes for enlargement, nodules, tenderness, or a gritty sensation. (See *A close look at the thyroid gland,* page 118.) Lowering the patient's chin slightly and turning toward the side you're palpating relaxes the muscle and may be helpful in your assessment.

Auscultating the neck

Finally, auscultate the neck. Using light pressure on the bell of the stethoscope, listen over the carotid arteries. Ask the patient to hold his breath while you listen, to prevent breath sounds from interfering with the sounds of circulation.

Listen for bruits, which signal turbulent blood flow. If you detected an enlarged thyroid gland, also auscultate the thyroid area with the bell. Check for a bruit or a soft rushing sound, which indicates a hypermetabolic state.

Abnormal findings

Common abnormalities you may find during an ear assessment include a perforated tympanic membrane, acute otitis media, carcinoma of the auricle, foreign bodies in the ear, and hearing loss. During a nose, mouth, and throat assessment, you may detect nasal flaring, nasal stuffiness

A close look at the thyroid gland

This illustration shows the structure and location of the thyroid gland.

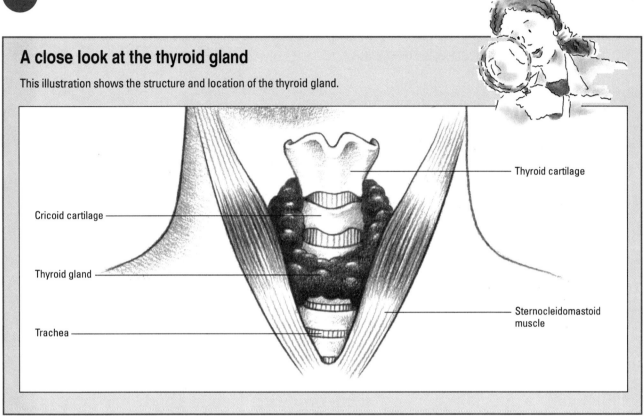

Thyroid cartilage

Cricoid cartilage

Thyroid gland

Trachea

Sternocleidomastoid muscle

and discharge, nasal pain, pharyngitis, and peritonsillar abscess.

Acute otitis media

More common in children than adults, acute otitis media causes the tympanic membrane to bulge and become inflamed.

Carcinoma of the auricle

A fairly common disorder, carcinoma of the auricle may be either basal cell or squamous cell. Advanced lesions are easy to diagnose, but small growths are often overlooked. Any crusted, indurated, or ulcerated lesion that fails to heal should be excised and examined.

Foreign bodies

Obstruction of the ear canal by a foreign body occurs most often in young children. Inanimate objects and vegetables are the most common objects found. Cotton is the most common foreign body found in the adult ear canal.

Pain and drainage may signal a foreign body, but sometimes no symptoms occur, and the object is found during a routine examination.

Hearing loss

Several factors can interfere with the ear's ability to conduct sound waves. The ear canal may be obstructed by a cerumen impaction, foreign body, or polyp. Otitis media can thicken the fluid in the middle ear, which interferes with the vibrations that transmit sound. Otosclerosis, a hardening of the bones in the middle ear, also interferes with the transmission of sound vibrations. Trauma can disrupt the middle ear's bony chain.

Sensorineural hearing loss also has several causes. (See *Evaluating hearing loss*, page 120.) The most common cause is loss of hair cells in the organ of Corti. In elderly people, presbycusis, or progressive hearing loss, results from atrophy of the organ or Corti and the auditory nerve. Hearing loss can also result from trauma to the hair cells caused by loud noise or ototoxicity.

In addition, drug toxicity can cause a rapid loss of hearing. If hearing loss is detected, the medication must be discontinued immediately. Drugs that may affect hearing include aspirin, aminoglycosides, loop diuretics, and several chemotherapeutic agents, including cisplatin.

Nasal flaring

Some nasal flaring is normal during quiet breathing in adults. It's also normal in children. Marked, regular nasal flaring in an adult may be a sign of respiratory distress.

Nasal stuffiness and discharge

Obstruction of the nasal mucous membranes along with a discharge of thin mucus can signal systemic disorders; nasal or sinus disorders such as a deviated septum; trauma, such as a basilar skull or nasal fracture; excessive use of vasoconstricting nose drops or sprays; and allergies or exposure to irritants, such as dust, tobacco smoke, or fumes. Nasal drainage accompanied by sinus tenderness and fever suggests acute sinusitis, which usually involves the frontal or maxillary sinuses.

Bloody discharge usually results from the patient blowing his nose, but spontaneous or traumatic epistaxis can also occur. Thick, white, yellow, or greenish drainage suggests an infection.

Evaluating hearing loss

Use this chart to review the causes, onset, and associated signs and symptoms of hearing loss.

Cause	Onset	Signs and symptoms
External ear		
Cerumen impaction	Sudden or gradual	Itching
Foreign body	Sudden	Discharge
Otitis externa	Sudden	Pain, discharge
Middle ear		
Serous otitis media	Sudden or gradual	Fullness, itching
Acute otitis media	Sudden	Pain, fever, upper respiratory tract infection
Perforated tympanic membrane	Sudden	Trauma, discharge
Inner ear		
Presbycusis	Gradual	None
Drug-induced loss	Sudden or gradual	Tinnitus, other adverse drug effects
Ménière's disease	Sudden	Dizziness
Acoustic neuroma	Gradual	Vertigo

Make sure to evaluate clear, thin drainage closely. It may simply indicate rhinitis, or it may be cerebrospinal fluid leaking from a basilar skull fracture.

Perforated tympanic membrane

A perforated tympanic membrane appears as a hole surrounded by reddened tissue. You may see discharge draining through the perforated area.

Peritonsillar abscess

Usually caused by acute tonsillitis, a peritonsillar abscess causes painful swallowing and a displaced, beefy, red uvula. It constitutes an emergency due to the potential for airway obstruction. In this condition, a streptococcal infection spreads from the tonsils to the surrounding soft tissue.

Pharyngitis

Discomfort in any part of the pharynx can range from scratchiness to severe pain. It can result from trauma, allergy, neoplasms, and certain systemic disorders.

Signs of viral pharyngitis are a slight swelling and inflammation of the pharynx. Streptococcal pharyngitis produces significant swelling and inflammation of the pharynx, exudate from the tonsils, and lymph node enlargement and tenderness. With infectious mononucleosis, the patient also has enlargement or tenderness of the cervical, inguinal, and axillary lymph nodes as well as exudative pharyngitis.

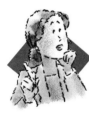

Quick quiz

1. Before inserting the otoscope into a patient's ear, the nurse should palpate the:
- A. helix.
- B. tragus.
- C. lymph nodes.

Answer: B. Before inserting the otoscope, palpate the tragus to make sure it's not tender. A tender tragus signals otitis externa.

2. During an otoscopic examination, the nurse should pull the superior posterior auricle of an adult patient's ear:
- A. up and back.
- B. up and forward.
- C. down and back.

Answer: A. In the adult patient, the superior posterior auricle should be pulled up and back to straighten the ear canal. In a child under age 3, pull the auricle down to get a good view of the membrane.

3. To assess the frontal sinuses, the nurse should palpate:
- A. on the forehead.
- B. below the cheekbones.
- C. over the temporal areas.

Answer: A. The frontal sinuses are located in the forehead, the site of palpation for those structures.

4. A cerumen impaction may contribute to a form of hearing loss called:
    A. central hearing loss.
    B. conductive hearing loss.
    C. sensorineural hearing loss.

Answer: B. Conductive hearing loss occurs from abnormal function of the external or middle ear, resulting in impaired sound transmission.

5. The patient's ability to identify a particular aroma depends on proper functioning of cranial nerve:
    A. I.
    B. II.
    C. IV.

Answer: A. Nasal patency and the olfactory nerve (cranial nerve I) are tested by having the patient identify an aroma.

Scoring

☆☆☆ If you answered all five items correctly, fantastic! You've won an all-expenses-paid trip to the sensational olfactory region!

☆☆ If you answered three or four correctly, excellent! You've won a cruise down the breathtaking nasal passage!

☆ If you answered fewer than three correctly, good work! You just won a gondola ride down the resoundingly resplendent ear canal!

Respiratory system

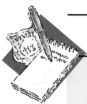

Just the facts

This chapter covers the respiratory system and how to assess problems associated with it. In this chapter, you'll learn:

♦ normal anatomy and physiology of the respiratory system

♦ how to assess the respiratory system using the four components of a physical examination

♦ abnormal findings for the respiratory system.

A look at the respiratory system

The respiratory system includes the airways, lungs, bony thorax, respiratory muscles, and central nervous system. (See *A close look at the respiratory system*, page 124.) They all work together to deliver oxygen to the bloodstream and remove excess carbon dioxide from the body. Knowing the basic structures and functions of the respiratory system will help you perform a comprehensive respiratory assessment and recognize any abnormalities.

Airways and lungs

The airways are divided into the upper and lower airways. The upper airways include the nasopharynx (nose), oropharynx (mouth), laryngopharynx, and larynx. Their purpose is to warm, filter, and humidify inhaled air. They also help to make sound and send air to the lower airways.

A close look at the respiratory system

The major structures of the upper and lower airways are illustrated below. The acinus is shown in the inset.

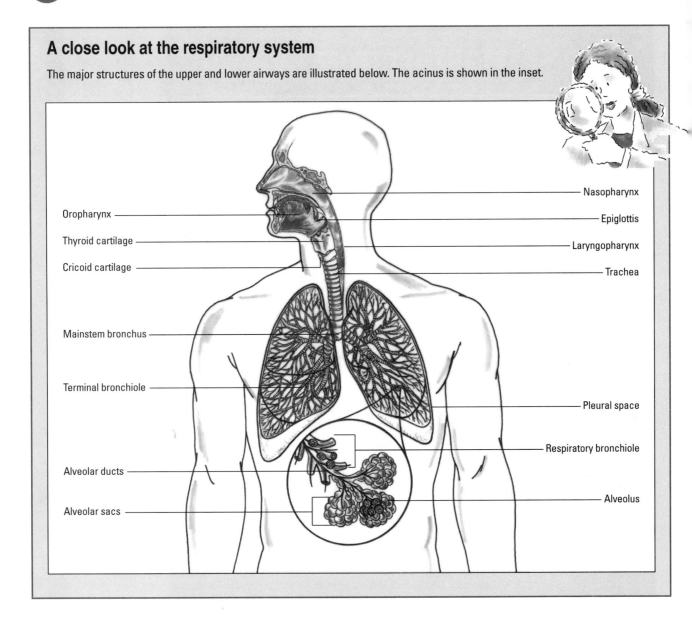

Oropharynx

Thyroid cartilage

Cricoid cartilage

Mainstem bronchus

Terminal bronchiole

Alveolar ducts

Alveolar sacs

Nasopharynx

Epiglottis

Laryngopharynx

Trachea

Pleural space

Respiratory bronchiole

Alveolus

The flap that protects

The epiglottis is a flap of tissue that closes over the top of the larynx when the patient swallows. The epiglottis protects the patient from aspirating food or fluid into the lower airways.

The larynx is located at the top of the trachea and houses the vocal cords. It's the transition point between the upper and lower airways.

The lowdown on the lower airways

The lower airways begin with the trachea, which then divides into the right and left mainstem bronchial tubes. The bronchial tubes divide into bronchi, which are lined with mucus-producing ciliated epithelium, one of the lungs' major defense systems.

The bronchi then divide into secondary bronchi, tertiary bronchi, terminal bronchioles, respiratory bronchioles, alveolar ducts and, finally, into the alveoli, the gas-exchange units of the lungs. The lungs in a typical adult contain about 300 million alveoli.

Lungs and lobes

Each lung is wrapped in a lining called the visceral pleura. The right lung is larger and has three lobes: upper, middle, and lower. The left lung is smaller and has only an upper and a lower lobe.

Smooth sliding

The lungs share space in the thoracic cavity with the heart and great vessels, the trachea, the esophagus, and the bronchi. The thoracic cavity is lined with parietal pleura in all areas that contact the lungs.

A small amount of fluid fills the area between the two layers of the pleura. That fluid, called pleural fluid, allows the layers of the pleura to slide smoothly over one another as the chest expands and contracts. The parietal pleura also contains nerve endings that give off pain signals when inflammation occurs.

Thorax

The bony thorax includes the clavicles, sternum, scapula, 12 sets of ribs, and 12 thoracic vertebrae. You can use specific parts of the thorax, along with some imaginary vertical lines drawn on the chest, to help describe the locations of your findings. (See *Respiratory assessment landmarks,* page 126.)

Ribs are made of bone and cartilage and allow the chest to expand and contract during each breath. All ribs attach to the vertebrae. The first seven ribs also attach directly to the sternum. The eighth and ninth ribs attach to the seventh rib. The eleventh and twelfth ribs are called floating ribs because they don't attach to anything in the front.

Respiratory muscles

The diaphragm and the external intercostal muscles are the primary muscles used in breathing. They contract when the patient inhales and relax when the patient exhales.

The respiratory center in the medulla initiates each breath by sending messages to the primary respiratory

Respiratory assessment landmarks

The illustration below shows common landmarks used in respiratory assessment.

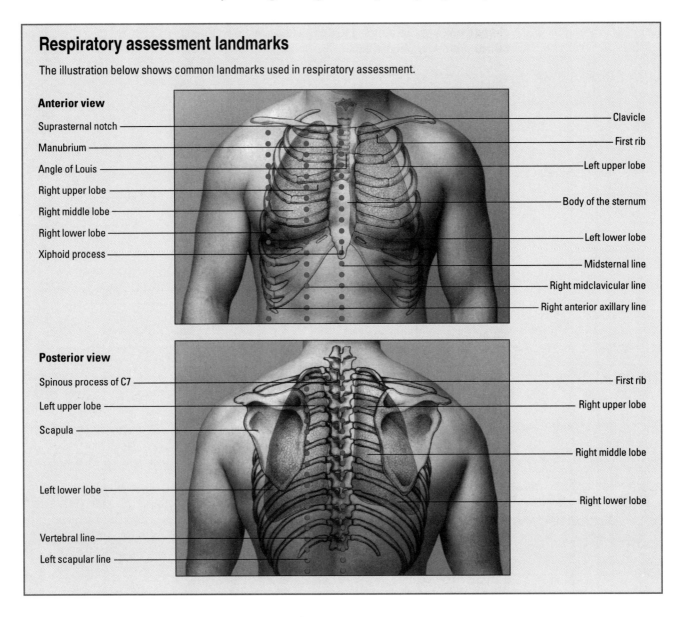

Anterior view

- Suprasternal notch
- Manubrium
- Angle of Louis
- Right upper lobe
- Right middle lobe
- Right lower lobe
- Xiphoid process

- Clavicle
- First rib
- Left upper lobe
- Body of the sternum
- Left lower lobe
- Midsternal line
- Right midclavicular line
- Right anterior axillary line

Posterior view

- Spinous process of C7
- Left upper lobe
- Scapula
- Left lower lobe
- Vertebral line
- Left scapular line

- First rib
- Right upper lobe
- Right middle lobe
- Right lower lobe

muscles over the phrenic nerve. (See *A close look at the mechanics of breathing.*) Impulses from the phrenic nerve adjust the rate and depth of breathing depending on the carbon dioxide and pH levels in the cerebrospinal fluid.

Accessory to breathing

Other muscles assist in breathing. Accessory inspiratory muscles include the trapezius, the sternocleidomastoid, and the scalenus, which combine to elevate the scapula, clavicle, sternum, and upper ribs. That elevation expands the front-to-back diameter of the chest when use of the diaphragm and intercostal muscles isn't effective.

Expiration occurs when the diaphragm and external intercostal muscles relax. If the patient has an airway obstruction, he may also use the abdominal muscles and internal intercostal muscles to exhale.

A close look at the mechanics of breathing

These illustrations show how mechanical forces, such as the movement of the diaphragm and intercostal muscles, produce a breath. A plus sign (+) indicates positive pressure, and a minus sign (-) indicates negative pressure.

At rest

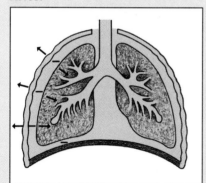

• Inspiratory muscles relax.
• Atmospheric pressure is maintained in the tracheobronchial tree.
• No air movement occurs.

Inhalation

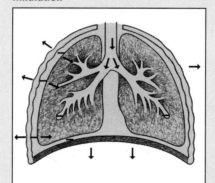

• Inspiratory muscles contract.
• The diaphragm descends.
• Negative alveolar pressure is maintained.
• Air moves into the lungs.

Exhalation

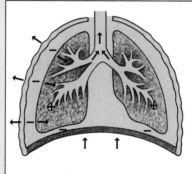

• Inspiratory muscles relax, causing lungs to recoil to their resting size and position.
• The diaphragm ascends.
• Positive alveolar pressure is maintained.
• Air moves out of the lungs.

Obtaining a health history

A patient with a respiratory disorder may complain of shortness of breath, cough, sputum production, wheezing, and chest pain (See *Breathtaking facts*.) Here are some helpful questions to gain information about each of those signs and symptoms.

Asking about shortness of breath

You can gain a history of shortness of breath by using several scales. Ask the patient to rate his usual level of dyspnea on a scale of 1 to 10, in which 1 means no dyspnea and 10 means the worst he has experienced. Then ask him to rate the level that day.

Other scales grade dyspnea as it relates to activity. In addition to one of the severity scales, you might also ask these questions: What do you do to relieve the dyspnea? How well does it work? (See *Grading dyspnea.*)

Asking about orthopnea

A patient with orthopnea (shortness of breath when lying down) tends to sleep with his upper body elevated. Ask this patient how many pillows he uses. The answer is then used to describe the severity of orthopnea. For instance, a patient who uses three pillows can be said to have "three-pillow orthopnea."

Asking about cough

Ask the patient with a cough these questions: Is the cough productive? If the cough is a chronic problem, has it changed recently? If so, how? What makes the cough better? What makes it worse?

Asking about sputum

When a patient produces sputum, ask him to estimate the amount produced in teaspoons or some other common measurement. At what time of day do you cough most often? What is the color and consistency of the sputum? If sputum is a chronic problem, has it changed recently? If so, how? Do you cough up blood? If so, how much and how often?

Asking about wheezing

If a patient wheezes, ask these questions: When does wheezing occur? What makes you wheeze? Do you

---

Breathtaking facts

Cough it up
• Coughing clears unwanted material from the tracheobronchial tree.
• Sputum from the bronchial tubes traps foreign matter and protects the lungs from damage.

Pain sites
The lungs themselves don't contain pain receptors, but chest pain may be caused by inflammation of the pleura or the costochondral joints at the midclavicular line or at the edge of the sternum.

How much O_2?
Patients with chronically high arterial carbon dioxide ($Paco_2$), such as those with COPD or a neuromuscular disease, may be stimulated to breathe by a low oxygen level (the hypoxic drive) rather than by a slightly high $Paco_2$ level, as is normal. For such patients, supplemental oxygen therapy should be provided cautiously. It may depress the stimulus to breathe, further increasing $Paco_2$.

wheeze loudly enough for others to hear it? What helps stop your wheezing?

Asking about chest pain

If the patient has chest pain, ask him these questions: Where is the pain located? What does it feel like? Is it sharp, stabbing, burning, or aching? Does it move to another area? How long does it last? What causes it to occur? What makes it better?

Chest pain that occurs from a respiratory problem is usually the result of pleural inflammation, inflammation of the costochondral junctions, soreness of chest muscles because of coughing, or indigestion. Less common causes of pain include rib or vertebral fractures caused by coughing or by osteoporosis.

Check the broader health history

Remember to look at the patient's medical and family history, being particularly watchful for a smoking habit, allergies, previous operations, and respiratory diseases, such as pneumonia and tuberculosis.

Be sure to ask about environmental exposure to irritants such as asbestos. (See *Listen and learn,* then *teach,* page 130.) People who work in mining, construction, or chemical manufacturing are often exposed to environmental irritants.

Assessing the respiratory system

Any patient can develop a respiratory disorder. By using a systematic assessment, you'll be able to detect subtle or obvious respiratory changes. The depth of your assessment will depend on several factors, including the patient's primary health problem and his risk of developing respiratory complications.

A physical examination of the respiratory system follows four steps: inspection, palpation, percussion, and auscultation. Before you begin, make sure the room is well lit and warm.

Make a few observations about the patient as soon as you enter the room. Note how the patient is seated, which will most likely be the position most comfortable for him. Take note of his level of awareness and general appearance. Does he appear relaxed? Anxious? Uncomfortable?

Grading dyspnea

To assess dyspnea as objectively as possible, ask your patient to briefly describe how various activities affect his breathing. Then document his response using the grading system.

Grade 0: not troubled by breathlessness except with strenuous exercise

Grade 1: troubled by shortness of breath when hurrying on a level path or walking up a slight hill

Grade 2: walks more slowly on a level path because of breathlessness than people of the same age or has to stop to breathe when walking on a level path at his own pace

Grade 3: stops to breathe after walking about 100 yards (91 m) on a level path

Grade 4: too breathless to leave the house or breathless when dressing or undressing

Is he having trouble breathing? You'll include those observations in your final assessment.

Inspecting the chest

Introduce yourself and explain why you're there. Help the patient into an upright position. The patient should be undressed from the waist up or clothed in an examination gown that allows you easy access to his chest.

Back, then front

Examine the back of the chest first, using inspection, palpation, percussion, and auscultation. Always compare one side with the other. Then examine the front of the chest using the same sequence. The patient can lie back when you examine the front of the chest if that's more comfortable for him.

Beauty in symmetry

Note masses or scars that indicate trauma or surgery. Look for chest wall symmetry. Both sides of chest should be equal at rest and expand equally as the patient inhales. The diameter of the chest, from front to back, should be about half the width of the chest.

In elderly patients, you may see a humpback appearance called kyphosis. This condition is caused by skeletal changes that occur with advanced age. In patients with kyphosis, the front-to-back diameter of the chest is increased.

A new angle

Also look at the angle between the ribs and the sternum at the point immediately above the xiphoid process. This angle — the costal angle — should be less than 90 degrees in an adult. The angle will be larger if the chest wall is chronically expanded because of an enlargement of the intercostal muscles, as can happen in chronic obstructive pulmonary disease (COPD).

Breathing rate and pattern

To find the patient's respiratory rate, count for a full minute — longer if you note abnormalities. Don't tell him what you're doing or he might alter his natural breathing pattern.

Adults normally breathe at a rate of 12 to 20 breaths/ minute. An infant's breathing rate may reach about 40

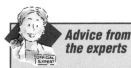

Advice from the experts

Listen and learn, *then* teach

Listening to what your patient says about his respiratory problems will help you know when he needs some patient education. The following typical responses indicate that the patient needs to know more about self-care techniques.

☑ "Whenever I feel breathless, I just take a shot of my inhaler." This patient needs to know more about proper use of an inhaler and when to call the doctor.

☑ "If I feel all congested, I just smoke a cigarette, and then I can cough up that phlegm!" This patient needs to know about the dangers of cigarette smoking.

☑ "None of the other guys wear a mask when we're working." This patient needs to know the importance of wearing an appropriate safety mask when working around heavy dust and particles in the air, such as sawdust or powders.

breaths/minute. (See *Types of breathing.*) The respiratory pattern should be even, coordinated, and regular, with occasional sighs. The ratio of inspiration to expiration (I:E) is about 1:2.

Raising a red flag

Watch for paradoxical, or uneven, movement of the chest wall. Paradoxical movement may appear as an abnormal collapse of part of the chest wall when the patient inhales or an abnormal expansion when the patient exhales. In either case, this uneven movement indicates a loss of normal chest wall function.

Muscles in motion

When the patient inhales, his diaphragm should descend and the intercostal muscles should contract. This dual motion causes the abdomen to push out and the lower ribs to expand laterally.

When the patient exhales, his abdomen and ribs return to their resting position. The upper chest shouldn't move much. Accessory muscles may hypertrophy, indicating frequent use. Frequent use of accessory muscles may be normal in some athletes, but for other patients it indicates a respiratory problem, particularly when the patient purses his lips and flares his nostrils when breathing.

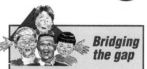

Bridging the gap

Types of breathing

In men, children, and infants, the most commonly used type of breathing is abdominal, or diaphragmatic, breathing. Athletes and singers also fall into that category. In most women, however, chest, or intercostal, breathing is used more often.

Inspecting related structures

Inspection of the skin, tongue, mouth, fingers, and nail beds may also provide information about respiratory status.

Skin color and nail beds

Skin color varies considerably among patients, but in all cases a patient with a bluish tint to his skin and mucous membranes is considered cyanotic. Cyanosis, which occurs when oxygenation to the tissues is poor, is a late sign of hypoxemia.

The most reliable place to check for cyanosis is the tongue and mucous membranes of the mouth. A chilled patient may have cyanotic nail beds, nose, or ears, indicating low blood flow to those areas but not necessarily to major organs.

Clubbing clues

When you check the fingers, look for clubbing, a possible sign of long-term hypoxia. A fingernail normally enters the skin at an angle of less than 180 degrees. When clubbing occurs, the angle is greater than or equal to 180 degrees.

Palpating the chest

Palpation of the chest provides some important information about the respiratory system and the processes involved in breathing. (See *Palpating the chest*.) Here's what to look for when palpating the chest.

No extra air

The chest wall should feel smooth, warm, and dry. Crepitus indicates subcutaneous air in the chest, an abnormal condition. Crepitus feels like puffed-rice cereal crackling under the skin and indicates that air is leaking from the airways or lungs.

Peak technique

Palpating the chest

To palpate the chest, place the palm of your hand (or hands) lightly over the thorax, as shown. Palpate for tenderness, alignment, bulging, or retractions of the chest and intercostal spaces. Assess for crepitus, especially around drainage sites. Repeat this procedure on the patient's back.

Next, use the pads of your fingers, as shown, to palpate the front and back of the thorax. Pass your fingers over the ribs and any scars, lumps, lesions, or ulcerations. Note the skin temperature, turgor, and moisture. Also note tenderness or bony or subcutaneous crepitus. The muscles should feel firm and smooth.

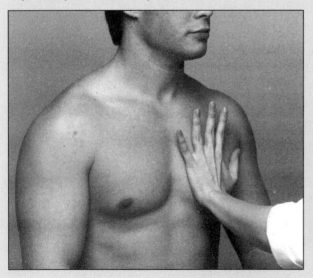
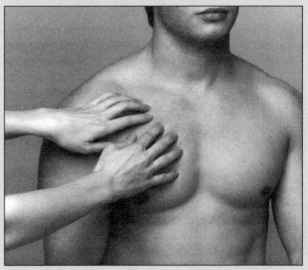

If a patient has a chest tube, you may find a small amount of subcutaneous air around the insertion site. If the patient has no chest tube or the area of crepitus is getting larger, alert the doctor immediately.

No pain

Gentle palpation shouldn't cause the patient pain. If the patient complains of chest pain, try to find a painful area on the chest wall. Painful costochondral joints are typically located at the midclavicular line or next to the sternum. Rib or vertebral fractures will be quite painful over the fracture, though pain may radiate around the chest as well. Pain may also be caused by sore muscles as a result of protracted coughing or a collapsed lung.

Vibratin' fremitus

Palpate for tactile fremitus, palpable vibrations caused by the transmission of air through the bronchopulmonary system. (See *Checking for tactile fremitus*.) Fremitus is decreased over areas where pleural fluid collects, when the patient speaks softly, and in pneumothorax, atelectasis, and

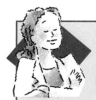

Peak technique

Checking for tactile fremitus

When you check the back of the thorax for tactile fremitus, ask the patient to fold his arms across his chest. This movement shifts the scapulae out of the way.

What to do
Check for tactile fremitus by lightly placing your open palms on both sides of the patient's back, as shown, without touching his back with your fingers. Ask the patient to repeat the phrase "ninety-nine" loud enough to produce palpable vibrations. Then palpate the front of the chest using the same hand positions.

What the results mean
Vibrations that feel more intense on one side than the other indicate tissue consolidation on that side. Less intense vibrations may indicate emphysema, pneumothorax, or pleural effusion. Faint or no vibrations in the upper posterior thorax may indicate bronchial obstruction or a fluid-filled pleural space.

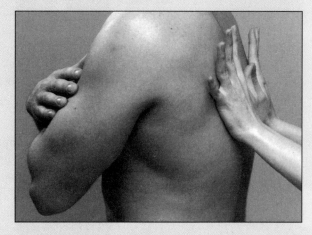

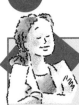

Peak technique

Percussing the chest

To percuss the chest, hyperextend the middle finger of your left hand if you're right-handed and the middle finger of your right hand if you're left-handed. Place your hand firmly on the patient's chest. Use the tip of the middle finger of your dominant hand — your right hand if you're right-handed, left hand if you're left-handed — to tap on the middle finger of your other hand just below the distal joint (as shown).

The movement should come from the wrist of your dominant hand, not your elbow or upper arm. Keep the fingernail you use for tapping short so you won't hurt yourself. Follow the standard percussion sequence over the front and back chest walls.

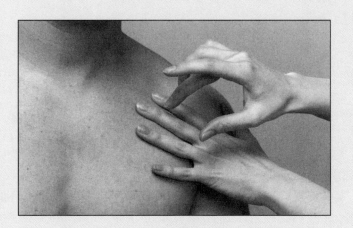

emphysema. Fremitus is increased normally over the large bronchial tubes and abnormally over areas in which alveoli are filled with fluid or exudate, as happens in pneumonia.

Measuring the symmetry

To evaluate the symmetry of the patient's chest wall and how much it expands, place your hands on the front of the chest wall, with your thumbs touching each other at the second intercostal space. As the patient inhales deeply, watch your thumbs. They should separate simultaneously and equally, to a distance several centimeters away from the sternum.

Repeat the measurement at the fifth intercostal space. The same measurement may be made on the back of the chest near the tenth rib.

Warning signs

The patient's chest may expand asymmetrically if he has pleural effusion, atelectasis, pneumonia, or pneumothorax. Chest expansion may be decreased at the level of the diaphragm if the patient has emphysema, respiratory depression, diaphragm paralysis, atelectasis, obesity, or ascites.

Percussing the chest

You'll percuss the chest to find the boundaries of the lungs; to determine whether the lungs are filled with air, fluid, or solid material; and to evaluate the distance the diaphragm travels between the patient's inhalation and exhalation . (See *Percussing the chest*.)

Different sites, different sounds

Percussion allows you to assess structures as deep as 3″ (7.6 cm). You'll hear different percussion sounds in different areas of the chest. (See *Percussion sounds*.)

You also may hear different sounds after certain treatments. For instance, if your patient has atelectasis and you percuss his chest before chest physiotherapy, you'll hear a high-pitched, dull, soft sound. After physiotherapy, you should hear a low-pitched, hollow sound. In all cases, make sure you use other assessment techniques to confirm percussion findings. (See *Double-check percussion findings*, page 136.)

What does it all mean?

Percussion sounds

Use this chart to help you become more comfortable with percussion and to quickly interpret percussion sounds. Learn the different percussion sounds by practicing on yourself, your patients, and any other person willing to help.

Sound	Description	Clinical significance
Flat	Short, soft, high-pitched, extremely dull, found over the thigh	Consolidation as in atelectasis and extensive pulmonary effusion
Dull	Medium in intensity and pitch, moderate length, thudlike, found over the liver	Solid area as in pleural effusion
Resonant	Long, loud, low-pitched, hollow	Normal lung tissue
Hyperresonant	Very loud, lower-pitched, found over the stomach	Hyperinflated lung as in emphysema or pneumothorax
Tympany	Loud, high-pitched, moderate length, musical, drumlike, found over a puffed-out cheek	Air collection as in a gastric air bubble or air in the intestines

Ringing with resonance

You'll hear resonant sounds over normal lung tissue, which you should find over most of the chest. In the left front chest, from the third or fourth intercostal space at the sternum to the third or fourth intercostal space at the midclavicular line, you should hear a dull sound. Percussion is dull here because that's the space occupied by the heart. Resonance resumes at the sixth intercostal space. The sequence of sounds in the back is slightly different. (See *Percussion sequences.*)

Problem sounds

When you hear hyperresonance during percussion, it means you've found an area of increased air in the lung or pleural space. Expect hyperresonance with pneumothorax, acute asthma, bullous emphysema (large holes in the lungs from alveolar destruction), and gastric distention that pushes up on the diaphragm.

When you hear abnormal dullness, it means you've found areas of decreased air in the lungs. Expect abnor-

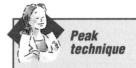

Peak technique

Double-check percussion findings

Use other assessment findings to verify the results of respiratory percussion. For example, if an X-ray report on a patient with chronic obstructive pulmonary disease indicates findings consistent with emphysema, you should hear low-pitched, loud, booming sounds when you percuss the chest.

Percussion sequences

Follow these percussion sequences to distinguish between normal and abnormal sounds in the patient's lungs. Remember to compare sound variations from one side with the other as you proceed. Carefully describe abnormal sounds you hear and include their locations. You'll follow the same sequences for auscultation.

Anterior

Posterior

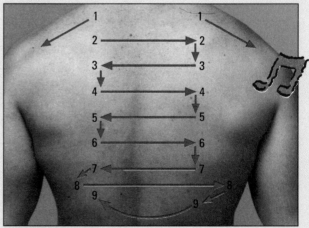

mal dullness in the presence of pleural fluid, consolidation, atelectasis, or a tumor.

Movement of the diaphragm

Percussion also allows you to assess how much the diaphragm moves during inspiration and expiration. The normal diaphragm descends 1¼″ to 3″ (3.2 to 7.6 cm) when the patient inhales. (See *Measuring diaphragm movement.*) The diaphragm doesn't move as far in patients with emphysema, respiratory depression, diaphragm paralysis, atelectasis, obesity, or ascites.

Auscultating the chest

As air moves through the bronchial tubes, it creates sound waves that travel to the chest wall. The sounds produced

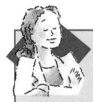

Peak technique

Measuring diaphragm movement

You can measure how much the diaphragm moves by first asking the patient to exhale. Percuss the back on one side to locate the upper edge of the diaphragm, the point at which normal lung resonance changes to dullness. Use a pen to mark the spot indicating the position of the diaphragm at full expiration on that side of the back.

Then ask the patient to inhale as deeply as possible. Percuss the back when the patient has breathed in fully until you locate the diaphragm. Use the pen to mark this spot as well. Repeat on the opposite side of the back.

Measure
Use a ruler or tape measure to determine the distance between the marks. The distance, normally 1¼″ to 2″ (3 to 5 cm) long, should be equal on both the right and left sides.

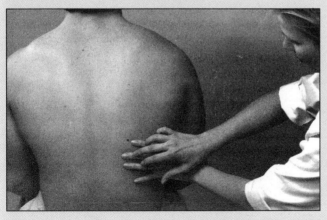

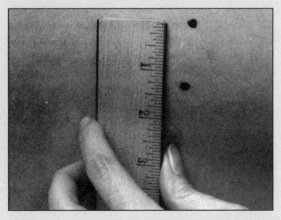

by breathing vary as air moves from larger airways to smaller airways. Sounds also change if they pass through fluid, mucus, or narrowed airways.

Auscultation helps you to determine the condition of the alveoli and surrounding pleura.

Preparing to auscultate

Auscultation sites are the same as percussion sites. Listen to a full inspiration and a full expiration at each site using the diaphragm of the stethoscope. Ask the patient to breathe through his mouth; nose breathing alters the pitch of breath sounds.

Quick tip: If the patient has abundant chest hair, mat it down with a damp washcloth so the hair doesn't make sounds like crackles.

Be firm

To auscultate for breath sounds, you'll press the stethoscope firmly against the skin. Remember that if you listen through clothing or dry chest hair, you may hear unusual and deceptive sounds.

Normal breath sounds

You'll hear four types of breath sounds over normal lungs. (See *Qualities of normal breath sounds*.) The type of sound you hear depends on where you listen. (See *Locations of normal breath sounds*.)

• Tracheal breath sounds are harsh, discontinuous sounds heard over the trachea. They occur when a patient inhales or exhales.

Qualities of normal breath sounds

Breath sound	Quality	Inspiration-expiration ratio	Location
Tracheal	Harsh, high-pitched	I < E	Over trachea
Bronchial	Loud, high-pitched	I > E	Next to trachea
Bronchovesicular	Medium in loudness and pitch	I = E	Next to sternum, between scapula
Vesicular	Soft, low-pitched	I > E	Remainder of lungs

• Bronchial breath sounds are loud, high-pitched sounds normally heard next to the trachea. They are discontinuous and are loudest when the patient exhales.

• Bronchovesicular sounds are medium-pitched, continuous sounds. They're heard when the patient inhales or exhales and are best heard over the upper third of the sternum and between the scapula.

• Vesicular sounds are soft, low-pitched sounds heard over the remainder of the lungs. They're prolonged when the patient inhales and shortened during exhalation.

What a change means

If you hear diminished but normal breath sounds in both lungs, the patient may have emphysema, atelectasis, severe bronchospasm, or shallow breathing. If breath sounds are heard in one lung only, the patient may have pleural effusion, pneumothorax, a tumor, or mucus plugs in the airways. In such cases, the doctor may order pulmonary function tests to further assess the patient's condition. (See *Interpreting pulmonary function test results,* page 140.)

Interpreting what you hear

Classify each sound according to its intensity, location, pitch, duration, and characteristic. Note whether the sound occurs when the patient inhales, exhales, or both. If you hear a sound in an area other than where you would expect to hear it, consider the sound abnormal.

For instance, bronchial or bronchovesicular breath sounds found in an area where vesicular breath sounds would normally be heard indicates that the alveoli and small bronchioles in that area might be filled with fluid or exudate, as happens in pneumonia and atelectasis. You won't hear vesicular sounds in those areas because no air is moving through the small airways.

The next step

A patient with abnormal findings during a respiratory assessment may be further evaluated using such diagnostic tests as arterial blood gas analysis or pulmonary function tests.

Vocal fremitus

Vocal fremitus is the sound produced by chest vibrations as the patient speaks. Abnormal transmission of voice sounds may occur over consolidated areas. Ask the patient to repeat the words listed below while you listen. Auscul-

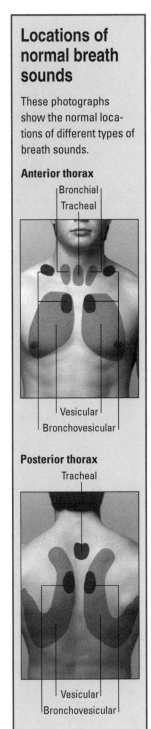

Locations of normal breath sounds

These photographs show the normal locations of different types of breath sounds.

Anterior thorax

Bronchial
Tracheal
Vesicular
Bronchovesicular

Posterior thorax

Tracheal
Vesicular
Bronchovesicular

What does it all mean?

Interpreting pulmonary function test results

You may need to interpret results of pulmonary function tests in your assessment of a patient's respiratory status. Use the chart below as a guide to common pulmonary function tests.

Restrictive and obstructive

The chart mentions restrictive and obstructive defects. A restrictive defect is one in which a person is unable to inhale a normal amount of air. It may occur with chest wall deformities, neuromuscular diseases, or acute respiratory infections.

An obstructive defect is one in which something obstructs the flow of air into or out of the lungs. It may occur with such diseases as asthma, chronic bronchitis, emphysema, or cystic fibrosis.

Test	Implications
Tidal volume (VT): amount of air inhaled or exhaled during normal breathing	Decreased VT may indicate restrictive disease and requires further tests, such as full pulmonary function studies or chest X-rays.
Minute volume (MV): amount of air breathed per minute	Normal MV can occur in emphysema. Decreased MV may indicate other diseases such as pulmonary edema.
Inspiratory reserve volume (IRV): amount of air inhaled after normal inspiration	Abnormal IRV alone doesn't indicate respiratory dysfunction. IRV decreases during normal exercise.
Expiratory reserve volume (ERV): amount of air that can be exhaled after normal expiration	ERV varies, even in healthy people.
Vital capacity (VC): amount of air that can be exhaled after maximum inspiration	Normal or increased VC with decreased flow rates may indicate reduction in functional pulmonary tissue. Decreased VC with normal or increased flow rates may indicate decreased respiratory effort, decreased thoracic expansion, or limited movement of the diaphragm.
Inspiratory capacity (IC): amount of air that can be inhaled after normal expiration	Decreased IC indicates restrictive disease.
Forced vital capacity (FVC): amount of air that can be exhaled after maximum inspiration	Decreased FVC indicates flow resistance in the respiratory system from obstructive disease, such as chronic bronchitis, emphysema, or asthma.
Forced expiratory volume (FEV): volume of air exhaled in the first (FEV_1), second (FEV_2), or third (FEV_3) FVC maneuver	Decreased FEV_1 and increased FEV_2 and FEV_3 may indicate obstructive disease. Decreased or normal FEV_1 may indicate restrictive disease.

tate over an area where you hear vesicular sounds and then again over an area where you hear bronchial breath sounds.

The presence of abnormal voice sounds — the most common of which are bronchophony, egophony, and whispered pectoriloquy — indicate the presence of consolidation. (See *Abnormal voice sounds.*)

Bronchophony. Ask the patient to say "ninety-nine" or "blue moon." Over normal lung tissue, the words sound muffled. Over consolidated areas, the words sound unusually loud.

Egophony. Ask the patient to say "E." Over normal lung tissue, the sound is muffled. Over consolidated lung tissue, it will sound like the letter *a*.

Whispered pectoriloquy. Ask the patient to whisper "1, 2, 3." Over normal lung tissue, the numbers will be almost indistinguishable. Over consolidated lung tissue, the numbers will be loud and clear.

Abnormal findings

Your assessment of the chest may reveal a number of abnormalities of the chest wall and lungs. Let's look first at chest wall abnormalities, which may be congenital or acquired. (See *Identifying chest deformities*, page 142.)

Chest wall abnormalities

As you examine a patient for chest wall abnormalities, keep in mind that patients with a deformity of the chest wall might have completely normal lungs and that the lungs might be cramped within the chest. The patient

---

Abnormal voice sounds

Bronchophony　　　　　**Egophony**　　　　　**Whispered pectoriloquy**

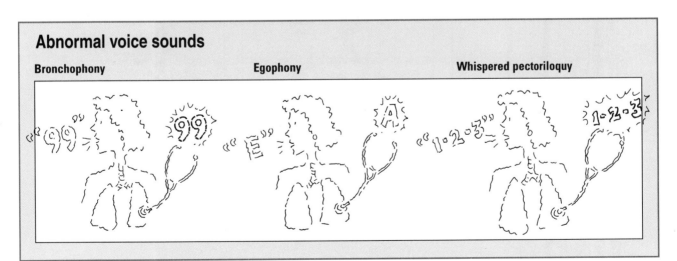

What does it all mean?

Identifying chest deformities

As you inspect the patient's chest, note deviations in size and shape. The illustrations here show a normal adult chest and four common chest deformities.

Normal adult chest

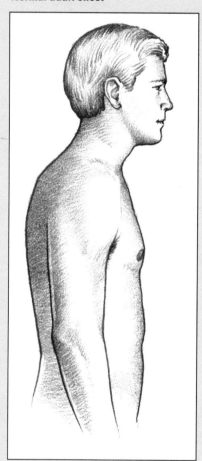

Barrel chest
Increased anteroposterior diameter

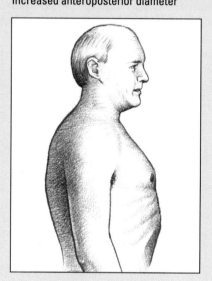

Funnel chest
Depressed lower sternum

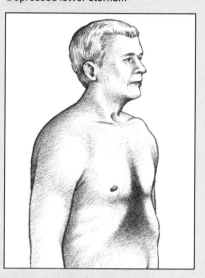

Pigeon chest
Anteriorly displaced sternum

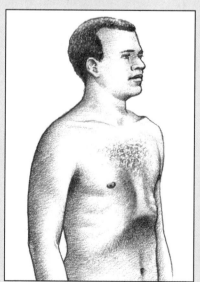

Thoracic kyphoscoliosis
Raised shoulder and scapula, thoracic convexity, and flared interspaces

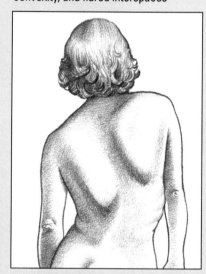

might have a smaller-than-normal lung capacity and limited exercise tolerance and he may more easily develop respiratory failure from a respiratory infection.

Barrel chest

A barrel chest looks like its name implies: The chest is abnormally round and bulging, with a greater-than-normal front-to-back diameter. Barrel chest may be normal in infants and elderly patients.

In other patients, barrel chest occurs as a result of COPD. In patients with COPD, barrel chest indicates that the lungs have lost their elasticity and that the diaphragm is flattened. You'll note that this patient typically uses accessory muscles when he inhales and easily becomes breathless. You'll also note kyphosis of the thoracic spine, ribs that run horizontally rather than tangentially, and a prominent sternal angle.

Pigeon chest

A patient with pigeon chest, or pectus carinatum, has a chest with a sternum that protrudes beyond the front of the abdomen. The displaced sternum increases the front-to-back diameter of the chest.

Funnel chest

A patient with funnel chest, or pectus excavatum, has a funnel-shaped depression on all or part of the sternum. The shape of the chest may interfere with respiratory and cardiac function. If cardiac compression occurs, you may hear a murmur.

Thoracic kyphoscoliosis

In this condition, the patient's spine curves to one side and the vertebrae are rotated. Because the rotation distorts lung tissues, you may have a more difficult time making a respiratory assessment.

Abnormal respiratory patterns

Identifying abnormal respiratory patterns can help you assess more completely a patient's respiratory status and his overall condition. (See *Spotting abnormal respiratory patterns*, page 144.)

Tachypnea

Tachypnea is a respiratory rate greater than 20 breaths/ minute with shallow breathing. It's often seen in patients with restrictive lung disease, pain, sepsis, obesity, and anx-

What does it all mean?

Spotting abnormal respiratory patterns

Here are typical characteristics of the more common abnormal respiratory patterns.

Tachypnea
Shallow breathing with increased respiratory rate

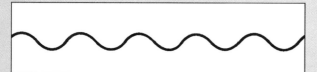

Bradypnea
Decreased rate but regular breathing

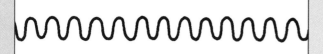

Apnea
Absence of breathing; may be periodic

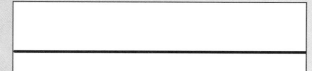

Hyperpnea
Deep breathing at a normal rate

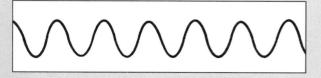

Kussmaul's respirations
Rapid, deep breathing without pauses; in adults, more than 20 breaths/minute; breathing usually sounds labored with deep breaths that resemble sighs

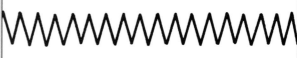

Cheyne-Stokes respirations
Breaths that gradually become faster and deeper than normal, then slower, during a 30- to 170-second period; alternates with 20- to 60-second periods of apnea

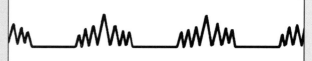

Biot's respirations
Rapid, deep breathing with abrupt pauses between each breath; equal depth to each breath

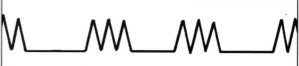

iety. Fever may be another cause. The respiratory rate may increase by 4 breaths/minute for every 1°F (0.6°C) rise in body temperature.

Bradypnea

Bradypnea is a respiratory rate below 10 breaths/minute and is often noted just before a period of apnea or full respiratory arrest. Patients with bradypnea might have central nervous system depression as a result of excessive sedation, tissue damage, or diabetic coma, which all depress the brain's respiratory control center. (The respiratory rate normally decreases during sleep.)

Apnea

Apnea is the absence of breathing. Periods of apnea may be short and occur sporadically during Cheyne-Stokes respirations, Biot's respirations, or other abnormal respiratory patterns. This condition may be life-threatening if periods of apnea last long enough.

Hyperpnea

Characterized by deep breathing, hyperpnea occurs in patients who exercise or who have anxiety, pain, or metabolic acidosis. In a comatose patient, hyperpnea may indicate hypoxia or hypoglycemia.

Kussmaul's respirations

Kussmaul's respirations are rapid, deep, sighing breaths that occur in metabolic acidosis, especially when associated with diabetic ketoacidosis.

Cheyne-Stokes respirations

Cheyne-Stokes respirations have a regular pattern of variations in the rate and depth of breathing. Deep breaths alternate with short periods of apnea. This respiratory pattern is seen in patients with congestive heart failure (CHF), kidney failure, or central nervous system damage. Cheyne-Stokes respirations may be normal during sleep in children and elderly patients.

Biot's respirations

Biot's respirations involve rapid deep breaths that alternate with abrupt periods of apnea. Biot's respirations are an ominous sign of severe central nervous system damage.

Abnormal breath sounds

Because solid tissue transmits sound better than air or fluid, breath sounds (as well as spoken or whispered words) will be louder than normal over areas of consolidation. If pus, fluid, or air fills the pleural space, breath sounds will be quieter than normal. If a foreign body or secretions obstruct a bronchus, breath sounds will be diminished or absent over lung tissue located distal to the obstruction.

Adventitious adventures

Adventitious sounds are abnormal no matter where you hear them in the lungs. Those sounds include fine and coarse crackles, wheezes, rhonchi, stridor, and pleural friction rub. (See *The latest word*.)

Crackles

Crackles are caused by collapsed or fluid-filled alveoli popping open. Heard primarily when the patient inhales, crackles are classified as either fine or coarse and usually don't clear with coughing. (See *Types of crackles*.)

Wheezes

Wheezes are high-pitched sounds heard first when a patient exhales. (See *When wheezing stops*.) The sounds occur when airflow is blocked. As severity of the block increases, wheezes may also be heard when the patient inhales. The sound of a wheeze doesn't change with coughing. Patients may wheeze as a result of asthma, infection, or CHF or when a tumor or foreign body obstructs the airways. (See *Signs of upper airway obstruction*, page 148.)

Rhonchi

Rhonchi are low-pitched, snoring, rattling sounds that occur primarily when a patient exhales, though they may also be heard when the patient inhales. Rhonchi usually change in sound or disappear with coughing. The sounds occur when fluid partially blocks the large airways.

Stridor

Stridor is a loud, high-pitched crowing sound that is heard (usually without a stethoscope) during inspiration and can usually be heard without a stethoscope. Stridor is caused by an obstruction in the upper airway and requires immediate attention.

The latest word

The terms used to describe adventitious breath sounds have changed over the years. You might still see or hear some of the terms listed here used in practice.

Crackles
Rales, crepitation

Wheezes
High-pitched wheezes, sibilant rhonchi

Rhonchi
Low-pitched or sonorous rhonchi

Types of crackles

Here's how to differentiate fine crackles from coarse crackles, a critical distinction when assessing the lungs.

Fine
These characteristics distinguish fine crackles:
- occur when the patient stops inhaling
- are usually heard in lung bases
- sound like a piece of hair being rubbed between the fingers or like Velcro being pulled apart
- occur in restrictive diseases, such as pulmonary fibrosis, asbestosis, silicosis, atelectasis, congestive heart failure, and pneumonia.

Coarse
These characteristics distinguish coarse crackles:
- occur when the patient starts to inhale; may be present when the patient exhales
- may be heard through the lungs and even at the mouth
- sound more like bubbling or gurgling, as air moves through secretions in larger airways
- occur in chronic obstructive pulmonary disease, bronchiectasis, pulmonary edema, and with severely ill patients who cannot cough; also called the "death rattle."

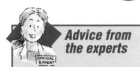

Advice from the experts

When wheezing stops

If you no longer hear wheezing in a patient having an acute asthma attack, the attack may be far from over. When bronchospasm and mucosal swelling become severe, little air can move through the airways. As a result, you won't hear wheezing.

If all other assessment criteria — labored breathing, prolonged expiratory time, accessory muscle use — point to acute bronchial obstruction, act to maintain the patient's airway and give oxygen, as ordered. The patient may begin wheezing again when the airways open more.

Pleural friction rub

Pleural friction rub is a low-pitched, grating, rubbing sound heard when the patient inhales and exhales. The rub is caused by pleural inflammation, which causes the two layers of pleura to rub together. The patient may complain of pain in areas where the rub is heard.

Respiratory disorders

Here's a list of specific respiratory disorders and the assessment findings you can expect.

Asthma

Asthma is a chronic disorder in which the airways are hyperreactive. The patient will have acute episodes of airway obstruction resulting from bronchospasm, increased mucus secretion, and mucosal edema.

Expect a sudden onset of dyspnea with increasing respiratory distress. You'll note wheezing, exhalation that takes longer than normal, and accessory muscle use. The patient may be anxious and may become cyanotic. You may detect vocal fremitus, diminished breath sounds, and hyperresonance in the lungs.

Atelectasis

A patient with atelectasis has a section of alveoli or an entire lung that has collapsed from airway obstruction, lack of surfactant (liquid in the alveoli), or compression of the chest wall. You may see decreased chest expansion on the affected side, an increased respiratory rate, dyspnea, cyanosis and, in severe cases, a shift of the trachea toward the affected side. You'll also note a lack of tactile fremitus over the area, dullness in percussion, and decreased or absent breath sounds.

Chronic bronchitis

In chronic bronchitis, changes in the tracheobronchial tree lead to inflammation, increased mucus production, ciliary damage, and blocked airways. Expect to see dyspnea, chronic cough with sputum production and tachypnea, and accessory muscle use. The lungs will be resonant, and you'll detect normal tactile fremitus. The patient may wheeze.

Emphysema

In a patient with emphysema, recurrent inflammation of the lungs destroys alveolar walls. Destruction of the alveoli creates large air spaces, decreases the elastic recoil of the lungs, and leads to trapped air and hyperinflated lungs.

Expect shortness of breath, a chronic cough, and possibly a barrel chest. The patient may breathe through pursed lips and use accessory muscles. His fingernails may be clubbed. Tactile fremitus and breath sounds will be decreased. Adventitious breath sounds, including wheezing, may vary.

Lobar pneumonia

In a patient with lobar pneumonia, an infection in the lungs causes fluid and cell debris to build up in the alveoli, which interferes with gas exchange. The patient will be tachypneic, possibly have pleuritic-type chest pain, sputum production, fever, and chills.

You may find dullness over the area and increased vocal fremitus. Also expect bronchial breath sounds and crackles over the affected area.

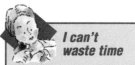
I can't waste time

Signs of upper airway obstruction

If a patient can't maintain a patent airway, he may end up in respiratory arrest. Refer to this list of potential signs and symptoms when assessing a patient for partial or complete airway obstruction:

• anxiety
• dyspnea
• stridor
• wheezes
• decreased or absent breath sounds
• use of accessory muscles
• seesaw movement between chest and abdomen
• inability to speak (complete obstruction)
• cyanosis.

Pleural effusion

In pleural effusion, fluid accumulates in the pleural space, making it difficult to hear breath sounds. The patient may be dyspneic and complain of pleuritic-type chest pain. In severe cases, the trachea may shift to the side opposite the effusion.

Chest expansion, tactile fremitus, and breath sounds may be decreased on the affected side. Percussion sounds may be dull or flat.

Pneumothorax

In a pneumothorax, air moves into pleural space and causes collapse of part or all of the lung. The severity of the patient's distress varies with the size of the pneumothorax. In any case, expect tachypnea, decreased chest wall expansion on the affected side, and possibly tracheal deviation away from the affected side. Tactile fremitus, vocal fremitus, and breath sounds will be decreased or absent over the area. Percussion will reveal hyperresonance.

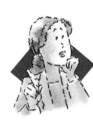

Quick quiz

1. In a patient with COPD, barrel chest indicates:
   A. loss of lung elasticity.
   B. rotation of the spinal column.
   C. increased elasticity of the intercostal muscles.

Answer: A. Barrel chest in patients with COPD is an indication of the loss of elasticity of the lungs and a flattening of the diaphragm. You'll also note accessory muscle use during inhalation and that the patient easily becomes breathless.

2. The percussion sound heard normally over most of the lungs is:
   A. dullness.
   B. resonance.
   C. hyperresonance.

Answer: B. The lungs are a mixture of lung tissue and air that makes a resonant percussion sound. Solid tissue is flat or dull; air-filled spaces are hyperresonant or tympanic.

3. To assess for hypoxemia, it's best to check for cyanosis of the:
    A. nail beds.
    B. facial skin.
    C. tongue and mucous membranes of the mouth.

Answer: C. Although cyanosis is a late sign of hypoxemia, it's best seen in the central mucous membranes, such as the tongue and mouth. Nail bed color is related more to perfusion rather than oxygenation.

4. Fine crackles are heard in:
    A. asthma.
    B. pulmonary fibrosis.
    C. neuromuscular disease.

Answer: B. Crackles are heard when collapsed or stiff alveoli snap open, as in pulmonary fibrosis. Wheezes are commonly associated with asthma and diminished breath sounds with neuromuscular disease.

5. When you auscultate the lower lobes of a healthy patient's lungs, you would expect to hear:
    A. tracheal breath sounds.
    B. bronchial breath sounds.
    C. vesicular breath sounds.

Answer: C. Vesicular breath sounds are soft, low-pitched, and prolonged during inspiration and can be heard over the lower lobes.

Scoring

☆☆☆ If you answered all five items correctly, excellent! You've left us breathless with your expertise!

☆☆ If you answered three or four correctly, hoorah! You're our resident respiratory guru!

☆ If you answered fewer than three correctly, no problem! You're first mate on our chest assessment team!

8

Cardiovascular system

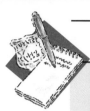

Just the facts

This chapter explains how to perform a complete cardiovascular assessment. In this chapter, you'll learn:

♦ about the structures that make up the cardiovascular system and how they function

♦ how to perform an assessment of the cardiovascular system

♦ how to tell the difference between normal and abnormal findings.

A look at the cardiovascular system

The cardiovascular system plays an important role in the body. It delivers oxygenated blood to tissues and removes waste products. The heart pumps blood to all organs and tissues of the body. The autonomic nervous system controls how the heart pumps. The vascular network — the arteries and veins — carries blood throughout the body, keeps the heart filled with blood, and maintains blood pressure. Let's look at each part of this critical system.

Heart

The heart is a hollow, muscular organ about the size of a closed fist. It's approximately 5″ (13 cm) long and 3 ½″ (9 cm) in diameter at its widest point. It weighs 1 to 1 ¼ lb (250 to 300 g). The heart is located between the lungs in the mediastinum, behind and to the left of the sternum.

Anatomy of the heart

The heart spans the area from the second to the fifth intercostal space. The right border of the heart lines up with the right border of the sternum. The left border lines up with the left midclavicular line. The exact position of the heart may vary slightly with each patient. Leading into and out of the heart are the great vessels: the inferior vena cava, the superior vena cava, the aorta, the pulmonary artery, and four pulmonary veins.

Smooth sliding

The heart is protected by a thin sac called the pericardium. The pericardium has an inner, or visceral, layer that forms the epicardium and an outer, or parietal, layer. The space between the two layers contains 10 to 30 ml of serous fluid, which prevents friction between the layers as the heart pumps.

Cardiac chambers

The heart has four chambers (two atria and two ventricles) separated by a cardiac septum. The upper atria have thin walls and serve as reservoirs for blood. They also boost the amount of blood moving into the lower ventricles, which fill primarily by gravity. (See *A close look at the heart.*)

Have blood, will travel

Blood moves to and from the heart through specific pathways. Deoxygenated venous blood returns to the right atrium through three vessels: the superior vena cava, inferior vena cava, and coronary sinus.

Blood from the upper body returns to the heart through the superior vena cava. Blood in the lower body returns through the inferior vena cava, and blood from the heart muscle itself returns through the coronary sinus. All of the blood from those vessels empties into the right atrium.

Into and through the heart

Blood in the right atrium empties into the right ventricle and is then ejected through the pulmonic valve into the pulmonary artery when the ventricle contracts. The blood then travels to the lungs to be oxygenated.

From the lungs, blood travels to the left atrium through the pulmonary veins. The left atrium empties the

A close look at the heart

This illustration details internal structures of the heart.

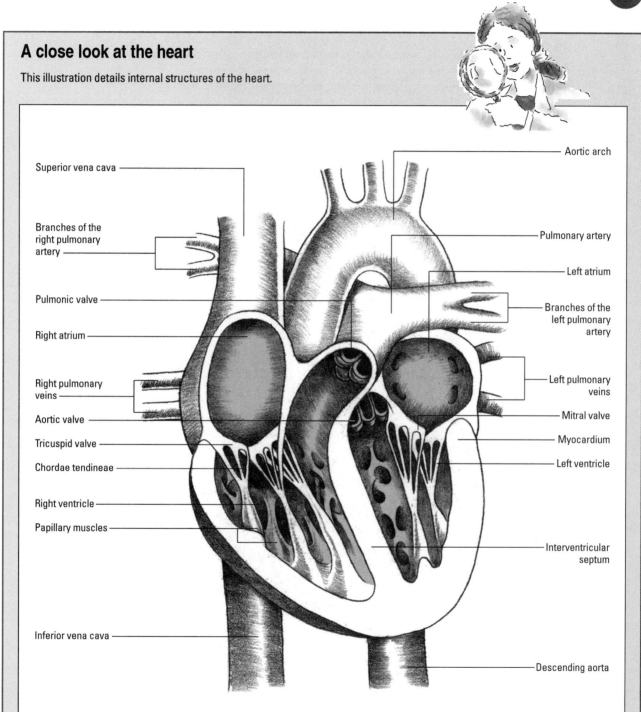

Superior vena cava

Branches of the
right pulmonary
artery

Pulmonic valve

Right atrium

Right pulmonary
veins

Aortic valve

Tricuspid valve

Chordae tendineae

Right ventricle

Papillary muscles

Inferior vena cava

Aortic arch

Pulmonary artery

Left atrium

Branches of the
left pulmonary
artery

Left pulmonary
veins

Mitral valve

Myocardium

Left ventricle

Interventricular
septum

Descending aorta

blood into the left ventricle, which then pumps the blood through the aortic valve into the aorta and throughout the body with each contraction. Because the left ventricle pumps blood against a much higher pressure than the right ventricle, its wall is three times thicker.

Valvular traffic cops

Valves in the heart keep blood flowing in only one direction through the heart. Think of the valves as traffic cops at the entrances to one-way streets, preventing blood from traveling the wrong way despite great pressure to do so. Healthy valves open and close passively as a result of pressure changes within the four heart chambers.

Which valve is where?

Valves between the atria and ventricles are called atrioventricular valves and include the tricuspid valve on the right side of the heart and the mitral valve on the left. Valves between the ventricles and the pulmonary vessels are called semilunar valves and include the pulmonic valve on the right and the aortic valve on the left.

Check out color pictures on pages 159 to 162.

On the cusp

Each valve's leaflets, or cusps, are anchored to the heart wall by cords of fibrous tissue. Those cords, called chordae tendineae, are controlled by papillary muscles. The cusps of the valves act to maintain tight closure. The tricuspid valve has three cusps. The mitral valve has two.

Physiology of the heart

Contractions of the heart occur in a rhythm — the cardiac cycle — and are regulated by impulses that normally begin at the sinoatrial (SA) node, the heart's pacemaker. The impulses are conducted from there throughout the heart. Impulses from the autonomic nervous system affect the SA node and alter its firing rate to meet the body's needs.

The cardiac cycle consists of systole, the period when the heart contracts and sends blood on its outward journey, and diastole, the period when the heart relaxes and fills with blood. During diastole, the mitral and tricuspid valves are open, and the aortic and pulmonic valves are closed.

Diastole: Parts I and II

Diastole consists of two parts, ventricular filling and atrial contraction. During the first part of diastole, 70% of the blood in the atria drains into the ventricles by gravity, a passive action.

The active period of diastole, atrial contraction (also called the atrial kick), accounts for the remaining 30% of blood that passes into the ventricles. Diastole is also the period in which the heart muscle receives its own supply of blood, transported there by the coronary arteries.

Of pressures, snaps, and sounds

Systole is the period of ventricular contraction. As pressure within the ventricles rises, the mitral and tricuspid valves snap closed. This closure leads to the first heart sound, S_1.

Once the pressure in the ventricles rises above the pressure in the aorta and pulmonary artery, the aortic and pulmonic valves open. Blood then flows from the ventricles into the pulmonary artery to the lungs and into the aorta to the rest of the body.

Cycle of life

At the end of ventricular contraction, pressure in the ventricles drops below the pressure in the aorta and the pulmonary artery. That pressure difference forces blood to back up toward the ventricles and causes the aortic and pulmonic valves to snap shut, which produces the second heart sound, S_2. As the valves shut, the atria fill with blood in preparation for the next period of diastolic filling, and the cycle begins again.

Vascular system

The peripheral vascular system consists of a network of arteries, arterioles, capillaries, venules, and veins that's constantly filled with about 5 L (10½ pints) of blood. (See *A close look at arteries and veins,* page 156.) The vascular system delivers oxygen, nutrients, and other substances to the body's cells and removes the waste products of cellular metabolism.

Thick-walled arteries

Arteries carry blood away from the heart. Nearly all arteries carry oxygen-rich blood from the heart throughout the

A close look at arteries and veins

This illustration shows major arteries and veins of the body.

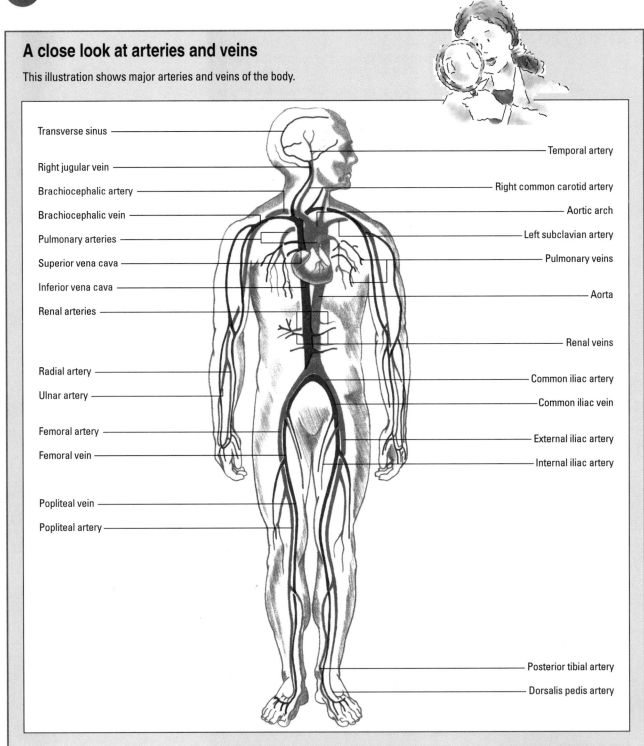

Transverse sinus

Right jugular vein

Brachiocephalic artery

Brachiocephalic vein

Pulmonary arteries

Superior vena cava

Inferior vena cava

Renal arteries

Radial artery

Ulnar artery

Femoral artery

Femoral vein

Popliteal vein

Popliteal artery

Temporal artery

Right common carotid artery

Aortic arch

Left subclavian artery

Pulmonary veins

Aorta

Renal veins

Common iliac artery

Common iliac vein

External iliac artery

Internal iliac artery

Posterior tibial artery

Dorsalis pedis artery

rest of the body. The only exception is the pulmonary artery, which carries oxygen-depleted blood to the lungs.

Arteries are thick-walled because they transport blood under high pressure. Arterial walls contain a tough, elastic layer to help propel blood through the arterial system.

Tiny capillaries

The exchange of fluid, nutrients, and metabolic wastes between blood and cells occurs in the capillaries. The exchange can occur because capillaries are thin-walled and highly permeable. Approximately 5% of the circulating blood volume at any given moment is contained within the capillary network. Capillaries are connected to arteries and veins through intermediary vessels called arterioles and venules, respectively.

Reservoir veins

Veins carry blood toward the heart. Nearly all veins carry oxygen-depleted blood, the sole exception being the pulmonary vein, which carries oxygenated blood from the lungs to the heart. Veins serve as a large reservoir for circulating blood.

The wall of a vein is thinner and more pliable than the wall of an artery. That pliability allows the vein to accommodate variations in blood volume. Veins contain valves at periodic intervals to prevent blood from flowing backward.

Pulses

Arterial pulses are pressure waves of blood generated by the pumping action of the heart. All vessels in the arterial system have pulsations, but the pulsations can be felt only where an artery lies near the skin. You can palpate for these peripheral pulses: carotid, radial, ulnar, brachial, femoral, popliteal, posterior tibial, dorsalis pedis, and temporal.

The location of pulse points varies between individuals. In older adults, peripheral pulses may be diminished.

Obtaining a health history

To obtain a health history of a patient's cardiovascular system, begin by introducing yourself and explaining what will occur during the health history and physical examination. Then obtain the following information.

Asking about the chief complaint

You'll find that patients with a cardiovascular problem often cite specific complaints, including:
- chest pain
- irregular heartbeat or palpitations
- shortness of breath on exertion, lying down, or at night
- cough
- cyanosis or pallor
- weakness
- fatigue
- unexplained weight change
- swelling of the extremities (see *Pregnancy and vein changes*)
- dizziness
- high or low blood pressure
- peripheral skin changes, such as decreased hair distribution, skin color changes, or a thin, shiny appearance to the skin
- pain in the extremities, such as leg pain or cramps.

Asking about personal and family health

Ask the patient for details not only about his chief complaint but also about his family history and past medical history, including diabetes or chronic diseases of the lungs, kidneys, or liver. (See *At risk for cardiovascular disease,* page 163.) Also obtain information about:
- previous operations
- stress levels and how he deals with them
- current health habits, such as smoking, alcohol intake, caffeine intake, exercise, and dietary intake of fat and sodium
- drugs the patient is currently taking, including over-the-counter drugs
- environmental or occupational considerations
- activities of daily living.

(Text continues on page 163.)

Pregnancy and vein changes

You might often find 4+ pitting edema in the legs of a pregnant patient in her third trimester. Severe edema is common not just in the third trimester but also in pregnant women who stand for long periods of time.

Varicose veins are another common finding in the third trimester.

Sites for heart sounds

When auscultating for heart sounds, place the stethoscope over the four different sites illustrated below.

Normal heart sounds indicate events in the cardiac cycle, such as the closing of heart valves, and are reflected to specific areas of the chest wall. Auscultation sites are identified by the names of heart valves, but they are not located directly over the valves. Rather, these sites are located along the pathway blood takes as it flows through the heart's chambers and valves.

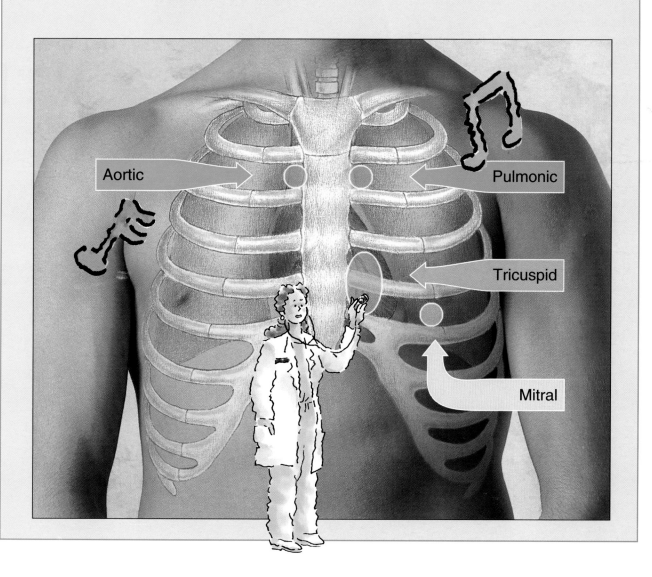

Aortic

Pulmonic

Tricuspid

Mitral

Cycle of heart sounds

When you auscultate a patient's chest and hear that familiar lub-dub, you're hearing the first heart sound, S_1, and the second heart sound, S_2. At times, two other sounds may occur normally: S_3 and S_4.

Heart sounds are generated by events in the cardiac cycle. When valves close or when blood fills the ventricles, vibrations of the heart muscle can be heard through the chest wall.

Varying sound patterns

The phonogram at right shows how heart sounds vary in duration and intensity. For instance, S_2 (which occurs when the semilunar valves snap shut) is a shorter-lasting sound than S_1 because the semilunar valves take less time to close than do the atrioventricular valves, which cause S_1.

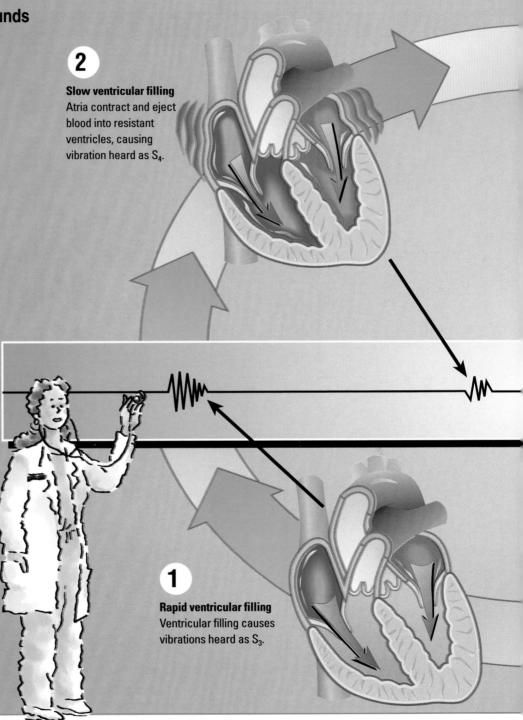

2

Slow ventricular filling
Atria contract and eject blood into resistant ventricles, causing vibration heard as S_4.

1

Rapid ventricular filling
Ventricular filling causes vibrations heard as S_3.

☐ Diastole

☐ Systole

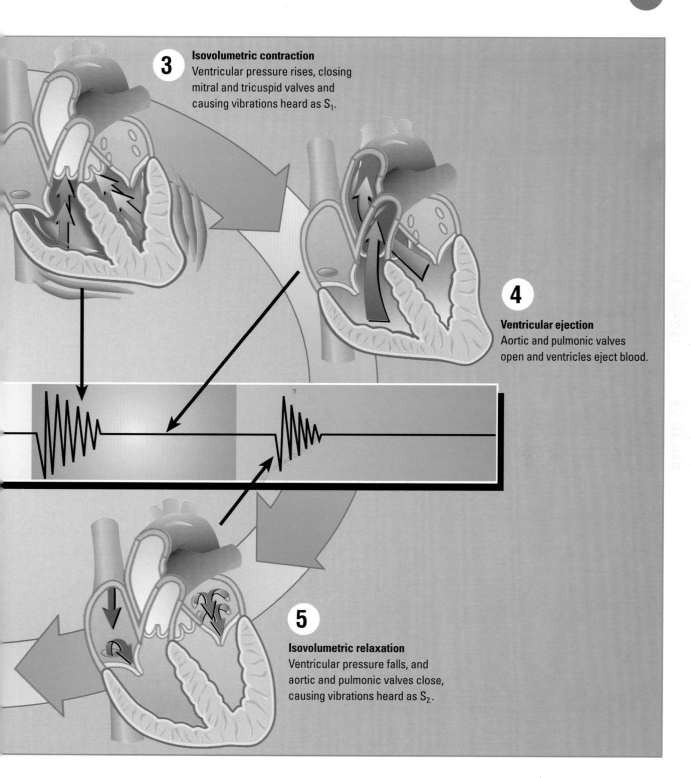

3 **Isovolumetric contraction**
Ventricular pressure rises, closing mitral and tricuspid valves and causing vibrations heard as S_1.

4 **Ventricular ejection**
Aortic and pulmonic valves open and ventricles eject blood.

5 **Isovolumetric relaxation**
Ventricular pressure falls, and aortic and pulmonic valves close, causing vibrations heard as S_2.

Understanding murmurs

Normally, heart valves close tightly and then open completely to let blood flow through. However, various conditions may alter blood flow through the valves, causing murmurs and, in many cases, increasing the workload of the heart.

The first two illustrations show a normal valve open and closed. The other illustrations portray three common reasons for the development of murmurs.

Normal valve open

Normal valve closed

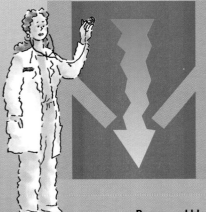

High blood flow
High blood flow through a normal valve may cause a murmur. Examples include an aortic systolic murmur, which can be caused by anemia and a subsequent compensatory increase in cardiac output.

Decreased blood flow
Low blood flow through a stenotic valve can cause a murmur. The valves can't open or close properly because they're thickened, fibrotic, or calcified. Common examples include aortic or mitral stenosis.

Backflow of blood
A backflow of blood through an insufficient or incompetent valve can cause a murmur. Because the valve can't close properly, blood can leak or regurgitate back into the heart chamber it came from. Common examples include aortic or mitral insufficiency.

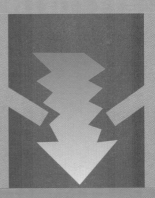

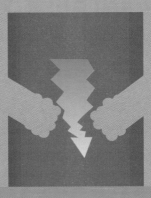

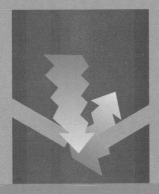

Rating the pain

Many patients with cardiovascular problems complain at some point of chest pain. (See *Understanding chest pain,* page 164.) If your patient has chest pain, ask him to rate the pain on a scale of 1 to 10, in which 1 means negligible and 10 means the worst he can imagine.

Asking about related problems

Besides checking for pain, also ask the patient these questions: Are you ever short of breath? If so, what activities cause you to be short of breath? Do you feel dizzy or fatigued? Do your rings or shoes feel tight? Do your ankles swell? Have you noticed changes in color or sensation in your legs? If so, what are those changes? If you have sores or ulcers, how quickly do they heal? Do you stand or sit in one place for long periods at work?

Assessing the cardiovascular system

Cardiovascular disease affects people of all ages and can take many forms. Using a consistent, methodical approach to your assessment will help you identify abnormalities. As always, the key to accurate assessment is regular practice, which will help improve technique and efficiency.

Before you begin your physical assessment, you'll need to obtain a stethoscope with a bell and a diaphragm, an appropriate-size blood pressure cuff, a ruler, and a penlight or other flexible light source. Make sure the room is quiet.

Ask the patient to remove all clothing except his underwear and to put on an examination gown. Have the patient lie on his back, with the head of the examination table at a 30- to 45-degree angle. Stand on the patient's right side if you're right-handed or left side if you're left-handed so you can auscultate more easily.

Assessing the heart

As with assessment of other body systems, you'll inspect, palpate, percuss, and auscultate in your assessment of the heart.

Bridging the gap

At risk for cardiovascular disease

As you analyze a patient's problems, remember that age, sex, and race are essential considerations in identifying patients at risk for cardiovascular disorders. For example, coronary artery disease most commonly affects white men between ages 40 and 60. Hypertension occurs most often in blacks.

Women are also vulnerable to heart disease, especially postmenopausal women and those with diabetes mellitus. Elderly people often have increased systolic blood pressure because of an increase in the rigidity of their blood vessel walls. Overall, aged people have a higher incidence of cardiovascular disease than younger people.

What does it all mean?

Understanding chest pain

Use this chart to help you more accurately assess chest pain.

What it feels like	Where it's located	What makes it worse	What causes it	What makes it better
Aching, squeezing, pressure, heaviness, burning pain; usually subside within 10 minutes	Substernal; may radiate to jaw, neck, arms, and back	Eating, physical effort, smoking, cold weather, stress, anger, hunger, lying down	Angina pectoris	Rest, nitroglycerin (*Note:* Unstable angina appears even at rest.)
Tightness or pressure; burning, aching pain; possibly accompanied by shortness of breath, diaphoresis, weakness, anxiety, or nausea; sudden onset; lasts ½ to 2 hours	Typically across chest but may radiate to jaw, neck, arms, or back	Exertion, anxiety	Acute myocardial infarction	Narcotic analgesics such as morphine sulfate
Sharp and continuous; may be accompanied by friction rub; sudden onset	Substernal; may radiate to neck or left arm	Deep breathing, supine position	Pericarditis	Sitting up, leaning forward, anti-inflammatory drugs
Excruciating, tearing pain; may be accompanied by blood pressure difference between right and left arm; sudden onset	Retrosternal, upper abdominal, or epigastric; may radiate to back, neck, or shoulders	Not applicable	Dissecting aortic aneurysm	Analgesics
Sudden, stabbing pain; may be accompanied by cyanosis, dyspnea, or cough with hemoptysis	Over lung area	Inspiration	Pulmonary embolus	Analgesics
Sudden and severe pain; sometimes accompanied by dyspnea, increased pulse rate, decreased breath sounds, or deviated trachea	Lateral thorax	Normal respiration	Pneumothorax	Analgesics, chest tube insertion
Dull, pressurelike, squeezing pain	Substernal, epigastric areas	Food, cold liquids, exercise	Esophageal spasm	Nitroglycerin, calcium channel blockers
Sharp, severe pain	Lower chest or upper abdomen	Eating a heavy meal, bending, lying down	Hiatal hernia	Antacids, walking, semi-Fowler's position
Burning feeling after eating sometimes accompanied by hematemesis or tarry stools; sudden onset that often subsides within 15 to 20 minutes	Epigastric	Lack of food or highly acidic foods	Peptic ulcer	Food, antacids
Gripping, sharp pain; possibly nausea and vomiting	Right epigastric or abdominal areas; possible radiation to shoulders	Eating fatty foods, lying down	Cholecystitis	Rest and analgesics, surgery
Continuous or intermittent sharp pain; possibly tender to touch; gradual or sudden onset	Anywhere in chest	Movement, palpation	Chest wall syndrome	Time, analgesics, heat applications
Dull or stabbing pain usually accompanied by hyperventilation or breathlessness; sudden onset; lasting less than a minute or as long as several days	Anywhere in chest	Increased respiratory rate, stress or anxiety	Acute anxiety	Slowing of respiratory rate, stress relief

Inspection

First, take a moment to assess the patient's general appearance. Is he overly thin? Obese? Alert? Anxious? Note his skin color, temperature, turgor, and texture. Are his fingers clubbed? (Clubbing is a sign of chronic hypoxia caused by a lengthy cardiovascular or respiratory disorder.) If the patient is dark-skinned, inspect his mucous membranes for pallor.

Checking out the chest

Next, inspect the chest. Note landmarks you can use to describe your findings, as well as structures underlying the chest wall. (See *Identifying cardiovascular landmarks.*)

Look for pulsations, symmetry of movement, retractions, or heaves. A heave is a strong outward thrust of the chest wall and occurs during systole.

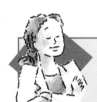

Peak technique

Identifying cardiovascular landmarks

These views show where to find critical landmarks used in cardiovascular assessment.

Anterior thorax

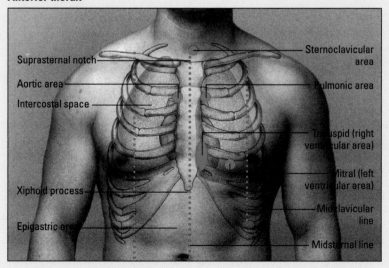

- Suprasternal notch
- Aortic area
- Intercostal space
- Xiphoid process
- Epigastric area
- Sternoclavicular area
- Pulmonic area
- Tricuspid (right ventricular area)
- Mitral (left ventricular area)
- Midclavicular line
- Midsternal line

Lateral thorax

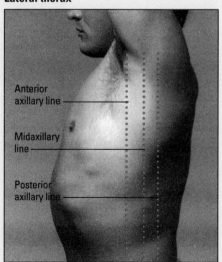

- Anterior axillary line
- Midaxillary line
- Posterior axillary line

Maximal impulse

Position a light source, such as a flashlight or gooseneck lamp, so that it casts a shadow on the patient's chest. Note the location of the apical impulse. This is also usually the point of maximal impulse and should be located in the fifth intercostal space medial to the left midclavicular line.

The apical impulse gives an indication of how well the left ventricle is working because it corresponds to the apex of the heart. The impulse can be seen in about 50% of adults. You'll notice it more easily in children and in patients with thin chest walls. To find the apical impulse in a woman with large breasts, displace the breasts during the examination.

Palpation

Maintain a gentle touch when you palpate so you won't obscure pulsations or similar findings. Using the ball of your hand, then your fingertips, palpate over the precordium to find the apical impulse. (See *Assessing the apical impulse.*) Note heaves or thrills, fine vibrations that feel like the purring of a cat.

The apical impulse may be difficult to palpate in obese patients and in patients with thick chest walls. If it's difficult to palpate with the patient lying on his back, have him lie on his left side or sit upright.

More areas to palpate

Also palpate the sternoclavicular, aortic, pulmonic, tricuspid, and epigastric areas for abnormal pulsations. Normally, you won't feel pulsations in those areas. An aortic arch pulsation in the sternoclavicular area or an abdominal aorta pulsation in the epigastric area may be a normal finding in a thin patient.

Percussing the heart

Although percussion isn't as useful as other methods of assessment, this technique may help you locate cardiac borders. Begin percussing at the anterior axillary line and percuss toward the sternum along the fifth intercostal space.

The sound changes from resonance to dullness over the left border of the heart, normally at the midclavicular line. The right border of the heart is usually aligned with the sternum and cannot be percussed.

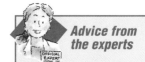

Advice from the experts

Assessing the apical impulse

The apical impulse is associated with the first heart sound and carotid pulsation. To ensure that you're feeling the apical impulse and not a muscle spasm or some other pulsation, use one hand to palpate the patient's carotid artery and the other to palpate the apical impulse. Then compare the timing and regularity of the impulses. The apical impulse should roughly coincide with the carotid pulsation.

Note the amplitude, size, intensity, location, and duration of the apical impulse. You should feel a gentle pulsation in an area about $1/2''$ to $3/4''$ (1.3 to 2 cm) in diameter.

Plumbing percussion problems

Percussion may be difficult in obese patients because of the fat overlying the chest or in female patients because of breast tissue. In this case, a chest X-ray can be used to provide information about the heart border.

Auscultating for heart sounds

You can learn a great deal about the heart by auscultating for heart sounds. Cardiac auscultation requires a methodical approach and lots of practice. Begin by warming the stethoscope in your hands, and then identify the sites where you'll auscultate: over the four cardiac valves and at Erb's point, the third intercostal space at the left sternal border. (See *Sites for heart sounds,* page 159.) Use the bell to hear low-pitched sounds and the diaphragm to hear high-pitched sounds.

Have a plan

Auscultate for heart sounds with the patient in three positions: lying on his back with the head of the bed raised 30 to 45 degrees, sitting up, and lying on his left side. (See *Auscultation tips.*) Use a zig-zag pattern over the precordium. You can start at the apex and work downward or at the base and work upward. Whichever approach you use, be consistent.

Use the diaphragm to listen as you go in one direction; use the bell as you come back in the other direction. Be sure to listen over the entire precordium, not just over the valves.

Note the heart rate and rhythm. Always identify S_1 and S_2, and then listen for adventitious sounds, such as S_3, S_4, murmurs, and rubs. (See *Cycle of heart sounds,* page 160 to 161.)

Listen for the "dub"

Start auscultating at the aortic area where S_2, the second heart sound, is loudest. S_2 is best heard at the base of the heart at the end of ventricular systole. The sound corresponds to closure of the pulmonic and aortic valves and is generally described as sounding like "dub." It's a shorter, higher-pitched, louder sound than S_1. When the pulmonic valve closes later than the aortic valve during inspiration, you'll hear a split S_2.

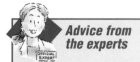

Advice from the experts

Auscultation tips

Follow these tips when you auscultate a patient's heart:

☑ Concentrate as you listen for each sound.

☑ Avoid auscultating through clothing or wound dressings because they can block sound.

☑ Avoid picking up extraneous sounds by keeping the stethoscope tubing off the patient's body and other surfaces.

☑ Until you gain proficiency at auscultation and can examine a patient quickly, explain to him that even though you may listen to his chest for a long period, it doesn't mean anything is wrong.

☑ Ask the patient to breathe normally and to hold his breath periodically to enhance sounds that may be difficult to hear.

Listen for the "lub"

From the base of the heart, move to the pulmonic area and then down to the tricuspid area. Then move to the mitral area, where S_1 is the loudest. S_1 is best heard at the apex of the heart. This sound corresponds to closure of the mitral and tricuspid valves and is generally described as sounding like "lub." It's low-pitched and dull. S_1 occurs at the beginning of ventricular systole. It may be split if the mitral valve closes just before the tricuspid.

S_3: Classic sign of CHF

A third heart sound, S_3, is frequently heard in children and in patients with a high cardiac output. Called ventricular gallop when it occurs in adults, S_3 may be a cardinal sign of congestive heart failure.

S_3 is best heard at the apex when the patient is lying on his back. Often compared to the *y* sound in "Ken-tuck-y," S_3 is low-pitched and occurs when the ventricles fill rapidly. It follows S_2 in early ventricular diastole and probably results from vibrations caused by abrupt ventricular distention and resistance to filling. Besides CHF, S_3 may also be associated with conditions such as pulmonary edema, atrial septal defect, and acute myocardial infarction (MI).

S_4: An MI aftereffect

S_4 is an adventitious sound called an atrial gallop that's heard over the tricuspid or mitral areas. You may hear S_4 in elderly patients or in patients with a previous MI. S_4, often described as sounding like "Ten-nes-see," occurs just before S_1, after atrial contraction.

The S_4 sound indicates increased resistance to ventricular filling. It results from vibrations caused by forceful atrial ejection of blood into ventricles that don't move or expand as much as they should.

Auscultating for murmurs

Murmurs occur when structural defects in the heart's chambers or valves cause turbulent blood flow. (See *Understanding murmurs,* page 162.) Turbulence may also be caused by changes in the viscosity of blood or the speed of blood flow. Listen for murmurs over the same precordial areas used in auscultation for heart sounds.

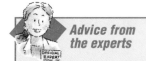

Advice from the experts

Tips for describing murmurs

Describing murmurs can be tricky. After you've auscultated a murmur, list the terms you would use to describe it. Then check the patient's chart to see how others have described it or ask an experienced colleague to listen and describe the murmur. Compare the descriptions, and then auscultate for the murmur again, if necessary, to confirm the description.

Check out color pictures on pages 159 to 162.

Murmur variations

Murmurs can occur during systole or diastole and are described by several criteria. (See *Tips for describing murmurs.*) Their pitch can be high, medium, or low. They can vary in intensity, growing louder or softer. (See *Grading murmurs.*) They can vary by location, sound pattern (blowing, harsh, or musical), radiation (to the neck or axillae), and period during which they occur in the cardiac cycle (pansystolic or midsystolic).

Sit up, please

The best way to hear murmurs is with the patient sitting up and leaning forward. (See *Positioning the patient for auscultation,* page 170.) You can also have him lie on his left side.

Auscultating for pericardial friction rub

Listening for a pericardial friction rub is also important. Have the patient sit upright, lean forward, and exhale. Listen with the diaphragm of the stethoscope over the third intercostal space on the left side of the chest. A pericardial friction rub has a scratchy, rubbing quality. *If you suspect a rub but have trouble hearing one, have the patient hold his breath.*

Assessing the vascular system

Assessment of the vascular system is an important part of a full cardiovascular assessment. Examination of the patient's arms and legs can reveal arterial or venous disorders. Examine the patient's arms when you take his vital signs. Check the legs later during the physical examination, when the patient is lying on his back. Remember to evaluate leg veins when the patient is standing.

Inspection

Start your assessment of the vascular system the same way you start an assessment of the cardiac system—by making general observations. Are the arms equal in size? Are the legs symmetrical?

Inspect the skin color. Note how body hair is distributed. Note lesions, scars, clubbing, and edema of the extremities. If the patient is confined to bed, be sure to

---

Grading murmurs

Use the system outlined below to describe the intensity of a murmur. When recording your findings, use Roman numerals as part of a fraction, always with VI as the denominator. For instance, a grade III murmur would be recorded as "grade III/VI."

- Grade I is a barely audible murmur.
- Grade II is audible but quiet and soft.
- Grade III is moderately loud, without a thrust or thrill.
- Grade IV is loud, with a thrill.
- Grade V is very loud, with a thrust or a thrill.
- Grade VI is loud enough to be heard before the stethoscope comes into contact with the chest.

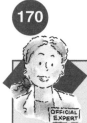

Advice from the experts

Positioning the patient for auscultation

If heart sounds are faint or undetectable, try listening to them with the patient seated and leaning forward or lying on his left side, which brings the heart closer to the surface of the chest. These illustrations show how to position the patient for high- and low-pitched sounds.

Leaning forward

The forward-leaning position is best suited for hearing high-pitched sounds related to semilunar valve problems, such as aortic and pulmonic valve murmurs. To auscultate for these sounds, place the diaphragm of the stethoscope over the aortic and pulmonic areas in the right and left second intercostal spaces, as shown.

Left lateral recumbent

The left lateral recumbent position is best suited for hearing low-pitched sounds, such as mitral valve murmurs and extra heart sounds. To hear these sounds, place the bell of the stethoscope over the apical area, as shown.

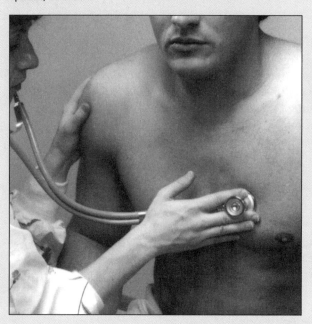

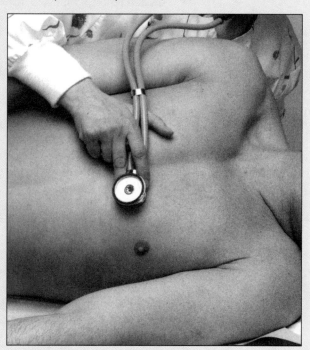

check the sacrum for swelling. Examine the fingernails and toenails for abnormalities.

Start at the top

Start your inspection by observing vessels in the neck. The carotid artery should appear as a brisk, localized pulsation. The internal jugular vein has a softer, undulating pulsation. The carotid pulsation doesn't decrease when the patient is upright, when he inhales, or when you palpate the carotid. The internal jugular pulsation, on the other hand, changes in response to position, breathing, and palpation.

Check carotid artery pulsations. Are they weak or bounding? Inspect the jugular veins. Inspection of these vessels can provide information about blood volume and pressure in the right side of the heart.

Checking on the jugular pulse

To check the jugular venous pulse, have the patient lie on his back. Elevate the head of the bed 30 to 45 degrees, and turn the patient's head slightly away from you. Normally, the highest pulsation occurs no more than 1½" (4 cm) above the sternal notch. If pulsations appear higher, it indicates central venous pressure and jugular vein distension.

Palpation

The first step in palpation is to assess skin temperature, texture, and turgor. Then check capillary refill by assessing the nail beds on the fingers and toes. Refill time should be no more than 3 seconds, or long enough to say "capillary refill."

Palpate the patient's arms and legs for temperature and edema. Edema is graded on a four-point scale. If your finger leaves a slight imprint, the edema is recorded as +1. If your finger leaves a deep imprint that only slowly returns to normal, the edema is recorded as +4.

Artery check!

Palpate for arterial pulses by gently pressing with the pads of your index and middle fingers. Start at the top of the patient's body at the temporal artery, and work your way down. Check the carotid, brachial, radial, femoral, popliteal, posterior tibial, and dorsalis pedis pulses.

Palpate for the pulse on each side, comparing pulse volume and symmetry. *Don't palpate both carotid arteries at the same time or press too firmly. If you do, the patient may faint or become bradycardic.* If you haven't put on gloves for the examination, do so when you palpate the femoral arteries.

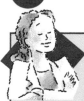

Peak technique

Assessing arterial pulses

To assess arterial pulses, apply pressure with your index and middle fingers. The following illustrations show where to position your fingers when palpating for various pulses.

Carotid pulse

Lightly place your fingers just medial to the trachea and below the jaw angle.

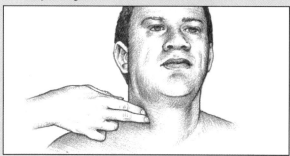

Brachial pulse

Position your fingers medial to the biceps tendon.

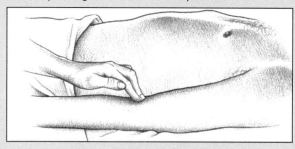

Radial pulse

Apply gentle pressure to the medial and ventral side of the wrist, just below the base of the thumb.

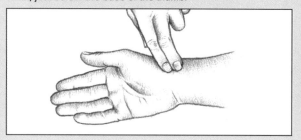

Femoral pulse

Press relatively hard at a point inferior to the inguinal ligament. For an obese patient, palpate in the crease of the groin, halfway between the pubic bone and the hip bone.

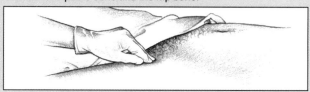

Popliteal pulse

Press firmly in the popliteal fossa at the back of the knee.

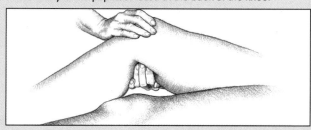

Posterior tibial pulse

Apply pressure behind and slightly below the malleolus of the ankle.

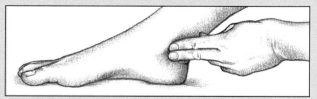

Dorsalis pedis pulse

Place your fingers on the medial dorsum of the foot while the patient points his toes down. The pulse is difficult to palpate here and may seem to be absent in healthy patients.

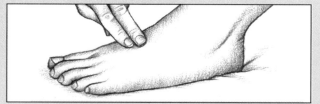

Grade that pulse!

All pulses should be regular in rhythm and equal in strength. (See *Assessing arterial pulses.*) Pulses are graded on the following scale: 4+ is bounding, 3+ is increased, 2+ is normal, 1+ is weak, and 0 is absent.

Auscultation

After you palpate, use the bell of the stethoscope to begin auscultation; then follow the palpation sequence and listen over each artery. You shouldn't hear sounds over the carotid arteries. A hum, or bruit, sounds like buzzing or blowing and could indicate arteriosclerotic plaque formation.

Assess the upper abdomen for abnormal pulsations, which could indicate the presence of an abdominal aortic aneurysm. Finally, auscultate for the femoral and popliteal pulses, checking for a bruit or other abnormal sounds.

Abnormal findings

This section outlines some of the more common abnormal findings from a cardiovascular system assessment and their causes.

Skin and hair abnormalities

Cyanosis, pallor, or cool or cold skin may indicate poor cardiac output and tissue perfusion. A number of conditions can cause fever or increased cardiac output and make the skin warmer than normal. Absence of body hair on the arms or legs may indicate diminished arterial blood flow to those areas. (See *Findings in arterial and venous insufficiency,* page 174.)

A cause for swelling

Swelling or edema may indicate CHF or venous insufficiency. They may also be caused by varicosities or thrombophlebitis.

Chronic right ventricular failure may cause ascites and generalized edema. If the patient has compression of a vein in a specific area, he may have localized swelling along the path of the compressed vessel. Right ventricular failure may cause swelling in the lower legs.

Abnormal pulsations

A displaced apical impulse may indicate an enlarged left ventricle, which may be caused by CHF or hypertension. A forceful apical impulse, or one lasting longer than a third of the cardiac cycle, may point to increased cardiac output. If you find a pulsation in the patient's aortic, pulmonic, or tricuspid area, his heart chamber may be enlarged or he may have valvular disease.

Pulses here, there, everywhere

Increased cardiac output or an aortic aneurysm may also produce pulsations in the aortic area. A patient with an epigastric pulsation may have early CHF or an aortic aneurysm. A pulsation in the sternoclavicular area sug-

---

Findings in arterial and venous insufficiency

Assessment findings differ in patients with arterial insufficiency and those with chronic venous insufficiency. These illustrations show those differences.

Arterial insufficiency

In a patient with arterial insufficiency, pulses may be decreased or absent. His skin will be cool, pale, and shiny and he may have pain in his legs and feet. Ulcerations often occur in the area around the toes, and the foot usually turns deep red when dependent. Nails may be thick and ridged.

Chronic venous insufficiency

In a patient with chronic venous insufficiency, check for ulcerations around the ankle. Pulses are present but may be difficult to find because of edema. The foot may become cyanotic when dependent.

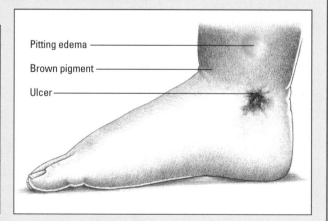

Pale, shiny skin

Thick, ridged nails

Redness

Ulcer

Pitting edema

Brown pigment

Ulcer

gests an aortic aneurysm. A patient with anemia, anxiety, increased cardiac output, or a thin chest wall might have slight pulsations to the right and left of the sternum.

Weak ones, strong ones

A weak arterial pulse may indicate decreased cardiac output or increased peripheral vascular resistance, both of which point to arterial atherosclerotic disease. Elderly patients often have weak pedal pulses.

Strong or bounding pulsations usually occur in patients with conditions that cause increased cardiac output, such as hypertension, hypoxia, anemia, exercise, or anxiety. (See *Pulse waveforms,* page 176.)

Thrills and heaves

A palpable thrill, or vibration, usually suggests a valvular dysfunction. A heave along the left sternal border may mean right ventricular hypertrophy; over the left ventricular area, a ventricular aneurysm.

Abnormal sounds

Abnormal auscultation findings include abnormal heart sounds (previously discussed), heart murmurs, and bruits. (See *Recognizing abnormal heart sounds,* page 177.)

Murmurs

Murmurs can occur as a result of a number of conditions and have widely varied characteristics. Here's a rundown on some of the more common murmurs.

Low-pitched murmur

Aortic stenosis, a condition in which the aortic valve has calcified and restricts blood flow, causes a midsystolic, low-pitched, harsh murmur that radiates from the valve to the carotid artery. The murmur shifts from crescendo to decrescendo and back.

Crescendo is a term used to describe the configuration of a murmur that increases in intensity. Likewise, a decrescendo murmur decreases in intensity. The crescendo-decrescendo murmur of aortic stenosis results from the turbulent, highly pressured flow of blood across stiffened leaflets and through a narrowed opening.

Advice from the experts

Pulse waveforms

To identify abnormal arterial pulses, check the waveforms below and see which one matches the patient's peripheral pulse.

Weak pulse

A weak pulse has a decreased amplitude with a slower upstroke and downstroke. Possible causes of a weak pulse include increased peripheral vascular resistance, such as happens in cold weather or severe congestive heart failure, and decreased stroke volume, as with hypovolemia or aortic stenosis.

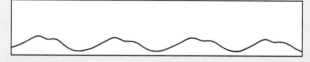

Bounding pulse

A bounding pulse has a sharp upstroke and downstroke with a pointed peak. The amplitude is elevated. Possible causes of a bounding pulse include increased stroke volume, as with aortic regurgitation, or stiffness of arterial walls, as with aging.

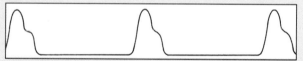

Pulsus alternans

Pulsus alternans has a regular, alternating pattern of a weak and a strong pulse. This pulse is associated with left ventricular failure.

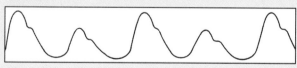

Pulsus bigeminus

Pulsus bigeminus is similar to pulsus alternans but occurs at irregular intervals. This pulse is caused by premature atrial or ventricular beats.

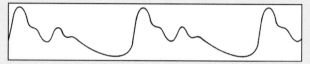

Pulsus paradoxus

Pulsus paradoxus has increases and decreases in amplitude associated with the respiratory cycle. Marked decreases occur when the patient inhales. Pulsus paradoxus is associated with pericardial tamponade, advanced heart failure, and constrictive pericarditis.

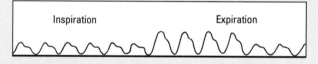

Pulsus biferiens

Pulsus biferiens shows an initial upstroke, a subsequent downstroke, and then another upstroke during systole. Pulsus biferiens is caused by aortic stenosis and aortic insufficiency.

Medium-pitched murmur

During auscultation, listen for a murmur near the pulmonic valve. This murmur might indicate pulmonic stenosis, a condition in which the pulmonic valve has calcified and interferes with the flow of blood out of the right ventricle. The murmur is medium-pitched, systolic, and harsh and shifts from crescendo to decrescendo and back. The

What does it all mean?

Recognizing abnormal heart sounds

Whenever auscultation reveals an abnormal heart sound, try to identify the sound and its timing in the cardiac cycle. Knowing those characteristics can help you identify the possible cause for the sound. Use this chart to put all that information together.

Abnormal heart sound	Timing	Possible causes
Accentuated S_1	Beginning of systole	Mitral stenosis, fever
Diminished S_1	Beginning of systole	Mitral regurgitation, heart block, or severe mitral regurgitation with a calcified, immobile valve
Split S_1	Beginning of systole	Right bundle-branch block
Accentuated S_2	End of systole	Pulmonary or systemic hypertension
Diminished or inaudible S_2	End of systole	Aortic or pulmonic stenosis
Persistent S_2 split	End of systole	Delayed closure of the pulmonic valve, usually from overfilling of the right ventricle, causing prolonged systolic ejection time
Reversed or paradoxical S_2 split that appears during expiration and disappears during inspiration	End of systole	Delayed ventricular stimulation, left bundle-branch block, or prolonged left ventricular ejection time
S_3 (ventricular gallop)	Early diastole	Overdistension of the ventricles during the rapid-filling segment of diastole or mitral insufficiency of ventricular failure (normal in children and young adults)
S_4 (atrial or presystolic gallop)	Late diastole	Pulmonic stenosis, hypertension, coronary artery disease, aortic stenosis, or forceful atrial contraction due to resistance to ventricular filling late in diastole (resulting from left ventricular hypertrophy)
Pericardial friction rub (grating or leathery sound at the left sternal border; usually muffled, high-pitched, and transient)	Throughout systole and diastole	Pericardial inflammation

murmur is caused by turbulent blood flow across a stiffened, narrowed valve.

High-pitched murmurs

In a patient with aortic insufficiency, the blood flows backward through the aortic valve and causes a high-pitched, blowing, decrescendo, diastolic murmur. The murmur radiates from the aortic valve area to the left sternal border.

In a patient with pulmonic insufficiency, the blood flows backward through the pulmonic valve, causing a blowing, diastolic, decrescendo murmur at Erb's point (at the left sternal border of the third intercostal space). If the patient has a higher than normal pulmonary pressure, the murmur is high-pitched. If not, it will be low-pitched.

Rumbling murmur

Mitral stenosis is a condition in which the mitral valve has calcified and is blocking blood flow out of the left atrium. Listen for a low-pitched, rumbling, crescendo-decrescendo murmur in the mitral valve area. This murmur results from turbulent blood flow across the stiffened, narrowed valve.

Blowing murmur

In a patient with mitral insufficiency, blood regurgitates into the left atrium. The regurgitation produces a high-pitched, blowing murmur throughout systole (pansystolic or holosystolic). The murmur may radiate from the mitral area to the left axillary line. You can hear it best at the apex.

Low, rumbling murmur

Tricuspid stenosis is a condition in which the tricuspid valve has calcified and is blocking blood flow through the valve from the right atrium. Listen for a low, rumbling, crescendo-decrescendo murmur in the tricuspid area. The murmur results from turbulent blood flow across the stiffened, narrowed valvular leaflets.

High-pitched, blowing murmur

In a patient with tricuspid insufficiency, blood regurgitates into the right atrium. This backflow of blood through the valve causes a high-pitched, blowing murmur throughout systole in the tricuspid area. The murmur becomes louder when the patient inhales.

Bruits

If you hear a bruit during arterial auscultation, the patient may have occlusive arterial disease or an arteriovenous fistula. Various high cardiac output conditions, such as anemia, hyperthyroidism, and pheochromocytoma, may also cause bruits.

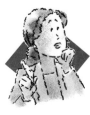

Quick quiz

1. When listening to heart sounds, you can hear S_1 best at the:
    A. base of the heart.
    B. apex of the heart.
    C. second intercostal space to the right of the sternum.

Answer: B. S_1 is best heard at the apex of the heart.

2. You are auscultating for heart sounds in a 3-year-old girl and hear an S_3. You assess this sound to be:
    A. a normal finding.
    B. a probable sign of CHF.
    C. a possible sign of atrial septal defect.

Answer: A. S_3 is a normal finding in a child. The sound can indicate CHF in an adult.

3. When grading arterial pulses, a 1+ grade pulse indicates:
    A. absent perfusion.
    B. diminished perfusion.
    C. normal perfusion.

Answer: B. A 1+ pulse indicates weak pulses and is associated with diminished cardiac perfusion.

4. You are assessing your client for jugular venous distention, so you would position him:
    A. sitting upright.
    B. flat on his back.
    C. lying on his back, with the head of the bed elevated 30 to 45 degrees.

Answer: C. Assessing jugular venous distention should be done when the patient is in semi-Fowler's position (head of the bed elevated 30 to 45 degrees). If the patient lies flat, the veins will be more distended; if he sits upright, the veins will be flat.

5. Capillary refill time is normally:
   A. 1 to 2 seconds.
   B. 3 to 5 seconds.
   C. 6 to 10 seconds.

Answer: A. Capillary refill time that's longer than 2 seconds is considered delayed and indicates decreased perfusion.

Scoring

☆☆☆ If you answered all five items correctly, take a bow! You're a star of the heart!

☆☆ If you answered three or four correctly, sensational! You're pumped with information!

☆ If you answered fewer than three correctly, keep at it! You're just getting the beat!

9

Breasts and axillae

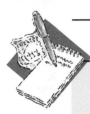

Just the facts

This chapter describes how to perform a complete assessment of the breasts and axillae in males and females. In this chapter you'll learn:

♦ what structures make up the breasts

♦ how the breasts change with age, pregnancy, and other conditions

♦ how to conduct a patient history about the breasts

♦ how to perform a physical assessment of the breasts and axillae

♦ what causes abnormalities of the breast and axillae—and how to recognize abnormalities.

A look at the breasts and axillae

With breast cancer becoming increasingly prominent in the news, more and more women are aware of the disease's risk factors, treatments, and diagnostic measures. By staying informed and performing breast self-examinations regularly, women can take control of their health and seek medical care when they notice a change in their breasts.

A matter of delicacy

No matter how informed a woman is, she can still feel anxious during breast examinations, even if she hasn't noticed a problem. That's because the social and psychological significance of the female breasts go far beyond their biological function. The breast is more than just a delicate structure; it's a delicate subject for women.

Keep this in mind during your assessment. It will help you to proceed carefully and professionally, so your patient feels more at ease.

Don't forget the men

Keep in mind that men also need breast examinations and that the incidence of breast cancer in males is rising. Men with breast disorders may feel uneasy or embarrassed about being examined because they see their conditions as being unmanly or a woman's problem. Remember that just as a woman needs a gentle, professional hand, so does a man.

Structures of the breast

The breasts, also called mammary glands in women, lie on the anterior chest wall. (See *The female breast.*) They're located vertically between the second or third and the sixth or seventh ribs over the pectoralis major muscle and the serratus anterior muscle, and horizontally between the sternal border and the midaxillary line.

Each breast has a centrally located nipple of pigmented erectile tissue ringed by an areola that's darker than the adjacent tissue. (See *Differences in areola pigmentation.*) Sebaceous glands, also called Montgomery's tubercles, are scattered on the areola surface, along with hair follicles.

The female breast

The illustration below shows a lateral cross section of the female breast.

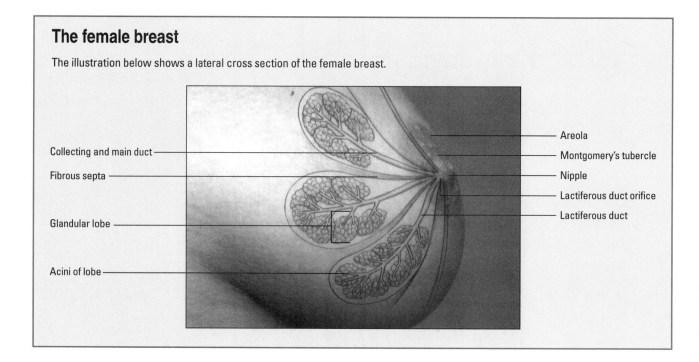

Collecting and main duct

Fibrous septa

Glandular lobe

Acini of lobe

Areola

Montgomery's tubercle

Nipple

Lactiferous duct orifice

Lactiferous duct

Support structures

Beneath the skin are glandular, fibrous, and fatty tissues that vary in proportion with age, weight, sex, and other factors such as pregnancy. A small triangle of tissue, called the tail of Spence, projects into the axilla. Attached to the chest wall musculature are fibrous bands called Cooper's ligaments that support each breast.

Lobes and ducts

In women, each breast is surrounded by 12 to 25 glandular lobes containing alveoli that produce milk. The lactiferous ducts from each lobe transport milk to the nipple. In men, the breast has a nipple, an areola, and mostly flat tissue bordering the chest wall.

Chains of draining nodes

The breasts also hold several lymph node chains, each serving different areas. The pectoral lymph nodes drain lymph fluid from most of the breast and anterior chest. The brachial nodes drain most of the arm. The subscapular nodes drain the posterior chest wall and part of the arm. The midaxillary nodes located near the ribs and the serratus anterior muscle high in the axilla are the central draining nodes for the pectoral, brachial, and subscapular nodes.

In women, the internal mammary nodes drain the mammary lobes. The superficial lymphatic vessels drain the skin. (See *Lymph node chains*, page 184.) In both men and women, the lymphatic system is the most common route of spread of cells that cause breast cancer.

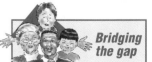

Bridging the gap

Differences in areola pigmentation

The pigment of the nipple and areola vary among different races, getting darker as skin tone darkens. Whites have light-colored nipples and areolae, usually pink or light beige. People with darker complexions, such as Blacks and Asians, have medium brown to almost black nipples and areolae.

How the breasts change with age

Women's breasts make many transformations throughout the life cycle. (See *Breast changes throughout life*, page 185.) Their appearance starts changing at puberty and continues changing during the reproductive years, pregnancy, and menopause.

Changes during puberty

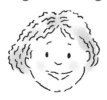

Thelarche, or breast development, is an early sign of puberty in girls. It usually occurs between ages 8 and 13. Menarche, the start of the menstrual cycle, typically occurs about 2 years later. Development of breast tissue in girls younger than age 8 is abnormal, and the patient should be referred to a doctor.

Lymph node chains

This illustration shows the different lymph node chains in the breast, axilla, and upper arm.

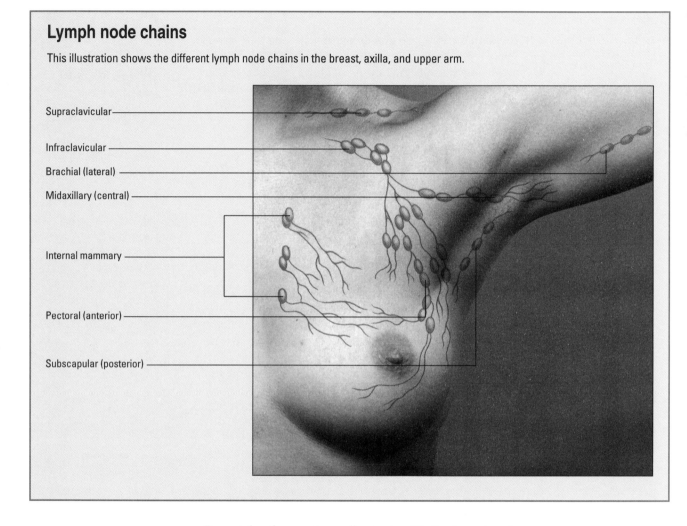

Supraclavicular

Infraclavicular

Brachial (lateral)

Midaxillary (central)

Internal mammary

Pectoral (anterior)

Subscapular (posterior)

Breast development usually starts with the breast and nipple protruding as a single mound of flesh. The shape of the adult female breast is formed gradually. During puberty, breast development is commonly unilateral or asymmetrical.

Breasts in boys

Young adolescent boys may have temporary stimulation of breast tissue due to the hormone estrogen, produced in both males and females. Breast enlargement in boys usually stops when they begin producing adequate amounts of the male sex hormone, testosterone.

Breast changes throughout life

The illustrations below show how a woman's breasts typically change from before puberty through menopause.

Before age 10

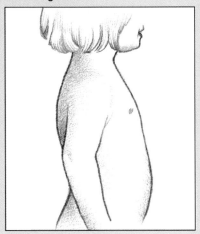

Between ages 10 and 14

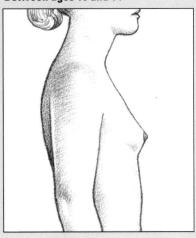

Adult woman who has never given birth

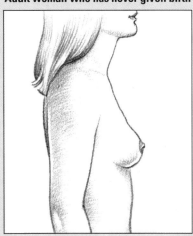

During pregnancy

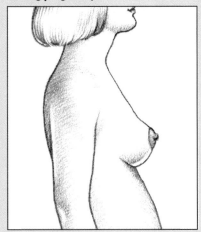

After pregnancy

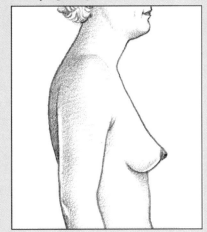

After menopause

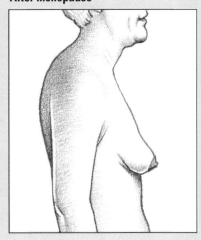

Changes during the reproductive years

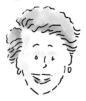

During the reproductive years, a woman's breasts may become full or tender in response to hormonal fluctuations during the menstrual cycle. During pregnancy, breast changes occur in response to hormones from the corpus luteum and the placenta.

The areola becomes deeply pigmented and increases in diameter. The nipple becomes darker, more prominent, and erect. The breasts enlarge due to the proliferation and hypertrophy of the alveolar cells and lactiferous ducts. As veins engorge, a venous pattern may become visible. In addition, striae may appear as a result of stretching, and Montgomery's tubercles may become prominent.

Changes after menopause

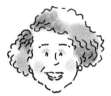

After menopause, estrogen levels decrease, causing glandular tissue to atrophy and be replaced with fatty deposits. The breasts become flabbier and smaller than they were before menopause. As the ligaments relax, the breasts hang loosely from the chest. The nipples flatten, losing some of their erectile quality. The ducts around the nipples may feel like firm strings.

Breasts in older men

Older men may have gynecomastia, or breast enlargement, due to age-related hormonal alterations or as an adverse effect of certain medications.

Obtaining a health history

Common complaints about the breasts include breast pain, nipple discharge and rash, and lumps, masses, and other changes. Complaints such as these — whether they come from women or men — warrant further investigation. (See *Evaluating breast lumps.*)

To investigate these complaints, ask about the symptom's onset, duration, and severity. For women, what day of the menstrual cycle do the symptoms appear? What relieves or worsens the symptoms?

Asking about past health

Ask the patient if she has ever had breast lumps, a breast biopsy, or breast surgery, including an enlargement or a reduction. If she has had breast cancer, fibroadenoma, or fibrocystic disease, ask for more information.

Inquire about her menstrual cycle, and record the date of her last period. If the patient has been pregnant, ask about the number of pregnancies and live births she has had. How old was she each time she became preg-

Evaluating breast lumps

If you find a breast lump during your assessment, evaluate it using this flowchart. Masses may be further investigated with a biopsy.

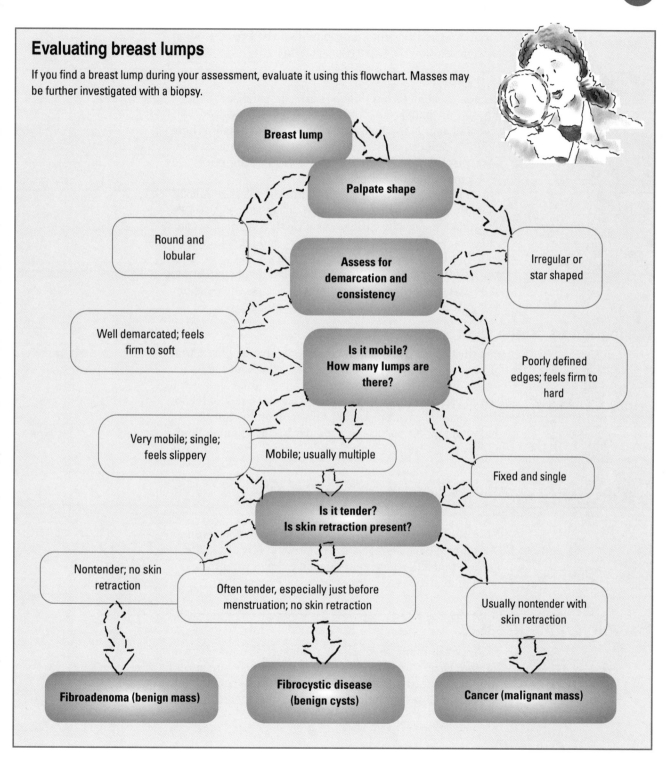

Breast lump

Palpate shape

Round and lobular

Assess for demarcation and consistency

Irregular or star shaped

Well demarcated; feels firm to soft

Is it mobile? How many lumps are there?

Poorly defined edges; feels firm to hard

Very mobile; single; feels slippery

Mobile; usually multiple

Fixed and single

Is it tender? Is skin retraction present?

Nontender; no skin retraction

Often tender, especially just before menstruation; no skin retraction

Usually nontender with skin retraction

Fibroadenoma (benign mass)

Fibrocystic disease (benign cysts)

Cancer (malignant mass)

nant? Did she have complications? Did she breast-feed or take medications to suppress lactation?

Asking about current health

Because certain breast changes are a normal part of aging, ask the patient how old she is. If she has noticed breast changes, ask her to describe them in detail. When did the changes occur? Does she have breast pain, tenderness, discharge, or rash? Has she noticed changes or problems in her underarm area?

Ask the patient what medications she takes regularly — birth control pills with estrogen, for instance. Also ask about diet, especially caffeine use. Birth control pills can cause breast swelling and tenderness, and ingestion of caffeine has been linked to fibrocystic disease of the breasts.

Ask the patient if she eats a high-fat diet, is under a lot of stress, smokes, or drinks alcohol. Discuss the possible link between those factors and breast cancer.

Asking about family health

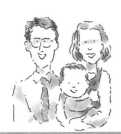

Ask the patient if any family members have had breast disorders, especially breast cancer. Also ask about the incidence of other types of cancer. Having a close relative with breast cancer greatly increases the patient's risk of having the disease. Teach the patient how to examine her breasts and about the importance of regular breast examinations and mammograms. (See *Scheduling breast examinations*.)

Assessing the breasts and axillae

Having a breast examination can be stressful for a woman. To reduce your patient's anxiety, provide privacy, make her as comfortable as possible, and explain what the examination involves.

Examining the breasts

Before examining the breasts, make sure the room is well lighted. Have the patient disrobe from the waist up and sit with her arms at her sides. Keep both breasts uncovered so you can observe them simultaneously to detect differences.

Scheduling breast examinations

The American Cancer Society and the American College of Radiology recommend the schedule shown below for regular breast examinations. Depending on their needs, some patients may follow a schedule modified by their doctor.

Age	Breast self-examination	Mammography	Physical examination
20 to 34	Monthly, 7 to 10 days after menstrual period begins	Not recommended	Every 3 years
35 to 39	Monthly, 7 to 10 days after menstrual period begins	One baseline mammogram within this time span	Every 3 years
40 to 50+	Monthly, 7 to 10 days after menstrual period begins (Postmenopausal women should examine their breasts on the same date each month. Have them pick a date that's significant to them, so they'll remember.)	Yearly	Yearly

Inspection

Observe the breast skin; it should be smooth, undimpled, and the same color as the rest of the skin. Check for edema, which can accompany lymphatic obstruction and may signal cancer. Note breast size and symmetry. Asymmetry may occur normally in some adult women, with the left breast usually larger than the right. Inspect the nipples, noting their size and shape. If a nipple is inverted (dimpled or creased), ask the patient when she first noticed the inversion.

Changing positions

Next, have the patient hold her arms over her head, and then with her hands on her hips, while you inspect the breasts. Having the patient assume these positions will help you detect skin or nipple dimpling that might not have been obvious before.

If the patient has large or pendulous breasts, have her stand with her hands on the back of a chair and lean forward. This position helps reveal subtle breast or nipple asymmetry.

Palpation

Before palpating the breasts, ask the patient to lie in a supine position, and place a small pillow under her shoulder on the side you're examining. This causes the breast on that side to protrude.

Then have the patient put her hand behind her head on the side you're examining. This spreads the breast more evenly across the chest and makes finding nodules easier. If her breasts are small, she can leave her arm at her side.

Compress and circle

To perform palpation, place your fingers flat on the breast and compress the tissues gently against the chest wall, palpating in concentric circles outward from the nipple. (See *Palpating the breast.*) Palpate the entire breast, including the periphery, tail of Spence, and areola. For patients with pendulous breasts, palpate down or across the breast with the patient sitting upright.

Watch for inconsistencies

As you palpate, note the consistency of the breast tissue. Normal consistency varies widely, depending in part on the proportions of fat and glandular tissue. Check for nodules and unusual tenderness. Remember: *Nodularity, fullness, and mild tenderness are premenstrual symptoms. Be sure to ask your patient where she is in her menstrual cycle.*

Tenderness may also be related to cysts and cancer. A lump or mass that feels different from the rest of the breast tissue may be a pathologic change and warrants further investigation by a doctor. If you find what you think is an abnormality, check the other breast, too. *Keep in mind that the inframammary ridge at the lower edge of the breast is normally firm and may be mistaken for a tumor.*

Documenting a mass

If you palpate a mass, record the following characteristics:
• size in centimeters
• shape — round, discoid, regular, or irregular
• consistency — soft, firm, or hard
• mobility
• degree of tenderness
• location, using the quadrant or clock method. (See *Identifying locations of breast lesions*, page 192.)

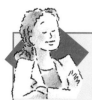

Peak technique

Palpating the breast

Use your three middle finger pads to palpate the breast systematically. Rotating your fingers gently against the chest wall, move in concentric circles. Make sure you include the tail of Spence in your examination.

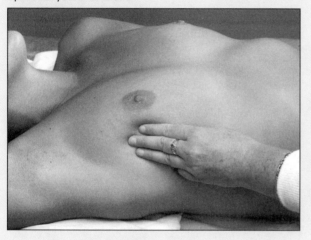

Examining the nipple

After palpating the breast, palpate the areola and nipple. Gently squeeze the nipple between your thumb and index finger to check for discharge.

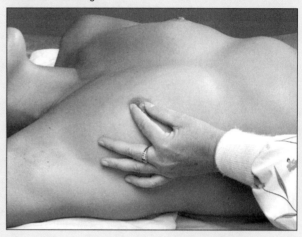

When to get a smear

Finally, palpate the nipple, noting its elasticity. It should be rough, elastic, and round. The nipple also typically protrudes from the breast. Compress the nipple and areola to detect discharge. If discharge is present and the patient isn't pregnant or lactating, assess the color, consistency, and quantity of the discharge. If possible, obtain a cytologic smear.

To obtain a smear, put on gloves, place a glass slide over the nipple, and smear the discharge on the slide. Spray the slide with a fixative, label it with the patient's name and date, and send it to the laboratory, according to your institution's policy.

Don't overlook palpation of the nipple and areola in male patients; assess for the same changes.

Examining the axillae

To examine the axillae, use the techniques of inspection and palpation. With the patient sitting or standing, inspect

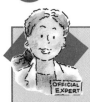

Advice from the experts

Identifying locations of breast lesions

Mentally divide the breast into four quadrants and a fifth segment, the tail of Spence. Then describe your findings according to the appropriate quadrant or segment. You can also think of the breast as a clock, with the nipple in the center. Then specify locations according to the time (2 o'clock, for example). Either way, specify the location of a lesion or other findings by the distance in centimeters from the nipple.

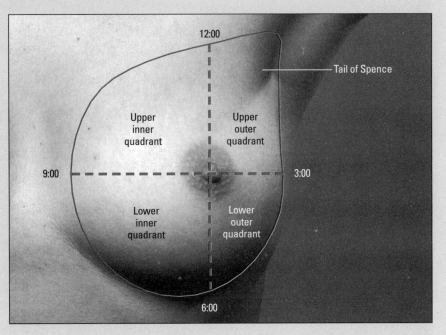

the skin of the axillae for rashes, infections, or unusual pigmentation.

Before palpating, ask the patient to relax her arm on the side you're examining. Support her elbow with one of your hands. (See *Palpating the axillae.*) Cup the fingers of your other hand, and reach high into the apex of the axilla. Place your fingers directly behind the pectoral muscles, pointing toward the midclavicle.

Assessing the axillary nodes

First, try to palpate the central nodes by pressing your fingers downward and in toward the chest wall. You can usually palpate one or more of the nodes, which should be soft, small, and nontender. If you feel a hard, large, or tender lesion, try to palpate the other groups of lymph nodes for comparison.

To palpate the pectoral and anterior nodes, grasp the anterior axillary fold between your thumb and fingers and palpate inside the borders of the pectoral muscles. Palpate the lateral nodes by pressing your fingers along the upper inner arm. Try to compress these nodes against the humerus. To palpate the subscapular or posterior nodes, stand behind the patient and press your fingers to feel the inside of the muscle of the posterior axillary fold.

Checking the neck nodes

If the axillary nodes appear abnormal, assess the nodes in the clavicular area. To do this, have the patient relax her neck muscles by flexing her head slightly forward. Stand in front of her and hook your fingers over the clavicle beside the sternocleidomastoid muscle. Rotate your fingers deeply into this area to feel the supraclavicular nodes.

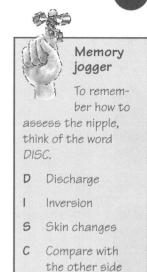

Memory jogger

To remember how to assess the nipple, think of the word DISC.

D   Discharge

I   Inversion

S   Skin changes

C   Compare with the other side

Abnormal findings

Because the menstrual cycle, certain prescription drugs, pregnancy, and other conditions can cause breast changes, you might have trouble differentiating abnormal changes from normal ones. To help you, the following section describes several common abnormal findings.

Peak technique

Palpating the axillae

To palpate the axillae, have the patient sit or lie down. Wear gloves if an ulceration or discharge is present. Ask her to relax her arm and then support it with your nondominant hand.

Keeping the fingers of your dominant hand together, reach high into the apex of the axillae, as shown. Position your fingers so they're directly behind the pectoral muscles, pointing toward the midclavicle. Sweep your fingers downward against the ribs and serratus anterior muscle to palpate the midaxillary or central lymph nodes.

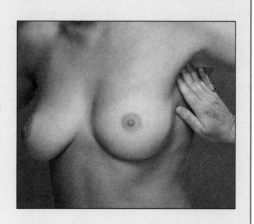

Fibrous breasts

In fibrocystic breasts, you may palpate one or more well-defined, moveable lumps or cysts. Fibrocystic disease is a benign condition that results from excess fibrous tissue formation and hyperplasia of the linings of the mammary ducts.

Fibroadenoma, also a benign condition, produces a small, round, painless, well-defined, mobile lump that may be soft but is usually solid, firm, and rubbery. (See *Dimpling and peau d'orange*.)

Malignant masses

A malignant breast mass may occur in any part of the breast, though it's usually found in the upper outer quadrant as a hard, immobile, irregular lump. Nipple discharge may occur, and breast skin may become edematous with enlarged pores, discoloration, and an orange-peel appearance.

Prominent breast veins

Prominent veins in the breast may indicate cancer in some patients but are normal in pregnant women due to engorgement.

Acute mastitis

Acute mastitis, or breast inflammation, causes reddening of the skin and abrasions or cracking. Fever and other signs of systemic infection may also occur. The condition is usually associated with lactation.

Paget's disease

Erythema of the nipple and areola may be an early sign of Paget's disease, a form of cancer of the mammary ducts. Nipple thickening, scaling, and erosion occur later. Another common sign of Paget's disease is a red, scaly, eczema-like rash over the affected nipple and areola.

Nipple and skin inversion

Inverted areas in the breast skin or nipple result from fibrosis or the formation of scar tissue and may be a sign of cancer. The breast or nipple may also change contour. Suspect fibrosis or cancer if inversion occurs suddenly with thickening or broadening of the skin. Keep in mind that inverted nipples may be normal if the patient has always had them.

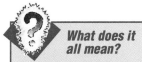

What does it all mean?

Dimpling and peau d'orange

These illustrations show two common abnormalities in breast tissue: dimpling and peau d'orange.

Dimpling
Dimpling usually suggests an inflammatory or malignant mass beneath the skin's surface. The illustration shows breast dimpling and nipple inversion caused by a malignant mass above the areola.

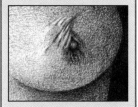

Peau d'orange
Peau d'orange is usually a late sign of breast cancer but it can also occur with breast or axillary lymph node infection. The skin's orange-peel appearance comes from lymphatic edema around deepened hair follicles.

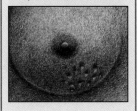

Male breast cancer and gynecomastia

Be aware that the incidence of male breast cancer has been increasing. Make sure to examine a man's breasts thoroughly during a complete physical assessment. Breast cancer in men usually occurs in the areolar area.

Gynecomastia is an abnormal enlargement of the male breast and may be caused by cirrhosis, leukemia, thyrotoxicosis, the administration of a hormone, or a hormonal imbalance.

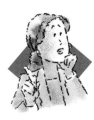

Quick quiz

1. Most malignant breast cancers occur in the region of the breast known as the:
- A. lower inner quadrant.
- B. lower outer quadrant.
- C. upper outer quadrant.

Answer: C. Although a malignancy can occur in any part of the breast, it usually occurs in the upper outer quadrant and appears as a hard, immobile, irregular lump.

2. Normal changes in the breasts of a premenstrual women include:
- A. a single hard, fixed mass.
- B. nipple inversion and skin dimpling.
- C. tenderness and soft, mobile cysts.

Answer: C. A week before menses, the breasts are usually tender with soft, benign, mobile, fluid-filled cysts in each breast.

3. After obtaining a smear of nipple discharge on a glass slide, you would:
- A. freeze the slide before sending it to the laboratory.
- B. let the smear air-dry before sending it to the laboratory.
- C. spray the slide with a cytologic fixative before sending it to the laboratory.

Answer: C. To obtain a culture of nipple discharge, place a glass slide over the nipple and smear the discharge on the slide. Then spray the slide with a cytologic fixative before sending it to the laboratory.

4. When her young son develops breast tissue, a mother asks you if the tissue will disappear soon. Your answer is based on the knowledge that breast enlargement in boys resolves when:

    A. the body produces adequate amounts of testosterone.

    B. the body produces adequate amounts of progesterone.

    C. the level of testosterone equals the level of progesterone.

Answer: A. When adequate amounts of the male sex hormone testosterone are produced, the effects of estrogen, including breast enlargement, decrease.

5. Tenderness, erythema, and swelling in one breast in a breast-feeding female probably indicates:

    A. mastitis.

    B. Paget's disease.

    C. normal engorgement.

Answer: A. The signs and symptoms listed indicate mastitis, an inflammation of breast tissues. Engorgement or overproduction or retention of breast milk can cause tenderness and swelling but usually not erythema.

6. The tail of Spence is located:

    A. in the lower outer quadrant, close to the ribs.

    B. in the upper inner quadrant, near the sternum.

    C. in the upper outer quadrant, toward the axilla.

Answer: C. The tail of Spence is a small triangle of tissue located in the upper outer quadrant of the breast, toward the axilla.

Scoring

☆☆☆ If you answered all six items correctly, way to go! You're an impeccable inspector and a palpator of prized precision!

☆☆ If you answered four or five correctly, good job! You're more than passable; you're a palpation ace!

☆ If you answered fewer than four correctly, that's okay! You're palpably poised on the edge of palpation greatness!

Gastrointestinal system

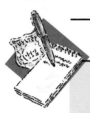

Just the facts

This chapter describes how to perform a full assessment of the various parts of the gastrointestinal (GI) system. In this chapter, you'll learn:

◆ what organs and structures make up the GI system

◆ how to obtain a patient history of the GI system

◆ how to perform a physical assessment of the GI system

◆ what conditions cause abnormalities in the GI system and how to recognize abnormalities.

A look at the GI system

The GI system's major functions include ingestion and digestion of food and elimination of waste products. When those processes are interrupted, the patient can experience problems ranging from loss of appetite to acid-base imbalances.

The GI system consists of two major divisions: the GI tract and the accessory organs. (See *Parts of the GI system, page 198.*)

GI tract

The GI tract is a hollow tube that begins at the mouth and ends at the anus. About 25′ (7.5 m) long, the GI tract consists of smooth muscle alternating with blood vessels and nerve tissue. Specialized circular and longitudinal fibers contract, causing peristalsis, which aids in propelling food through the GI tract. The GI tract includes the pharynx, esophagus, stomach, small intestine, and large intestine.

Parts of the GI system

This illustration shows the GI system's major anatomic structures. Knowledge of these structures will help you conduct an accurate physical assessment.

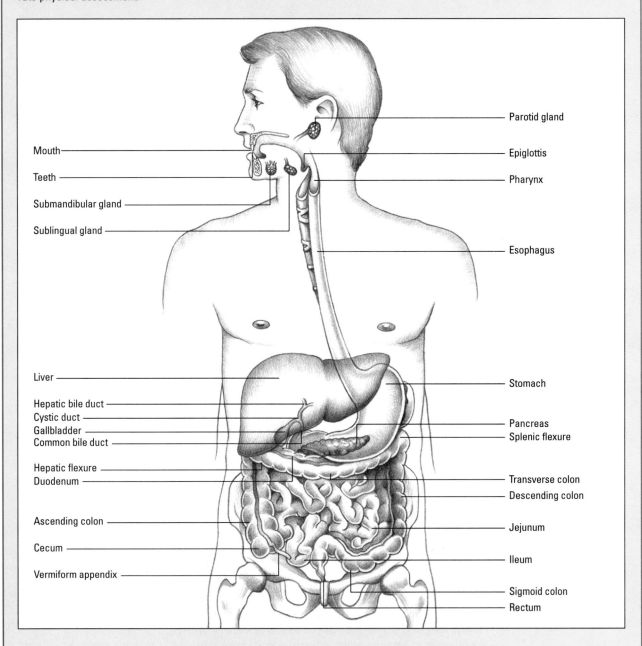

Mouth

Teeth

Submandibular gland

Sublingual gland

Parotid gland

Epiglottis

Pharynx

Esophagus

Liver

Hepatic bile duct
Cystic duct
Gallbladder
Common bile duct

Hepatic flexure
Duodenum

Ascending colon

Cecum

Vermiform appendix

Stomach

Pancreas
Splenic flexure

Transverse colon
Descending colon

Jejunum

Ileum

Sigmoid colon
Rectum

Start at the mouth

Digestive processes begin in the mouth with chewing, salivating, and swallowing. The tongue provides the sense of taste. Saliva is produced by three pairs of glands: the parotid, submandibular, and sublingual.

Proceed to the pharynx

The pharynx, or throat, allows the passage of food from the mouth to the esophagus. The pharynx assists in the swallowing process and secretes mucus that aids in digestion. The epiglottis, a thin, leaf-shaped structure made of fibrocartilage, is directly behind the root of the tongue. When food is swallowed, the epiglottis closes over the larynx and the soft palate lifts to block the nasal cavity. Those actions keep food and fluid from being aspirated into the airway.

Down the esophagus

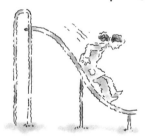

The esophagus is a muscular, hollow tube that moves food from the pharynx to the stomach. When food is swallowed, the upper esophageal sphincter relaxes, and the food moves into the esophagus. Peristalsis then propels the food toward the stomach. The gastroesophageal sphincter at the lower end of the esophagus normally remains closed to prevent reflux of gastric contents. The sphincter opens during swallowing, belching, and vomiting.

Stay awhile in the stomach

The stomach, a reservoir for food, is a dilated, saclike structure that lies obliquely in the left upper quadrant below the esophagus and diaphragm, to the right of the spleen, and partly under the liver. The stomach contains two important sphincters: the cardiac sphincter, which protects the entrance to the stomach, and the pyloric sphincter, which guards the exit.

The stomach has three major functions. It:
• stores food
• mixes food with gastric juices
• passes chyme — a watery mixture of partly digested food and digestive juices — into the small intestine for further digestion and absorption.

An average meal can remain in the stomach for 3 to 4 hours. Rugae, accordion-like folds in the stomach lining, allow the stomach to expand when large amounts of food and fluid are ingested.

Slip through the small intestine

The small intestine is 20′ (6 m) long and is named for its diameter, not its length. It has three sections: the duodenum, the jejunum, and the ileum. As food passes into the small intestine, the end products of digestion are absorbed through its thin mucous membrane lining into the bloodstream.

Carbohydrates, fats, and proteins are broken down in the small intestine. Secretions that aid digestion are enzymes from the pancreas, bile from the liver, and hormones from glands of the small intestine. These secretions mix with the food as it moves through the intestines. Food passes through the small intestine by peristalsis.

And finally head through the large intestine

The large intestine, or colon, is about 5′ (1.5 m) long and is responsible for:
• absorbing excess water and electrolytes
• storing food residue
• eliminating waste products in the form of feces.

The large intestine includes, in this order, the cecum; the ascending, transverse, descending, and sigmoid colons; the rectum; and the anus. The appendix, a fingerlike projection, is attached to the cecum. Bacteria in the colon produce gas or flatus.

Accessory organs

Accessory GI organs include the liver, pancreas, gallbladder, and bile ducts. The abdominal aorta and the gastric and splenic veins also aid digestion.

Look at the liver

The liver is located in the right upper quadrant under the diaphragm. It has two major lobes, divided by the falciform ligament.

The liver's functions include:
• metabolizing carbohydrates
• detoxifying blood
• converting ammonia to urea for excretion

• synthesizing plasma proteins, nonessential amino acids, vitamin A, and essential nutrients, such as iron and vitamins D, K, and B_{12}.

The liver also secretes bile, a greenish fluid that helps digest fats and absorb fatty acids, cholesterol, and other lipids. Bile also gives stool its color.

Gape at the gallbladder

The gallbladder is a small, pear-shaped organ that lies halfway under the right lobe of the liver. Its main function is to store bile from the liver until the bile is emptied into the duodenum. The emptying process occurs when the small intestine initiates chemical impulses that cause the gallbladder to contract.

Probe the pancreas

The pancreas lies horizontally in the abdomen, behind the stomach. It consists of a head, tail, and body. The body of the pancreas is located in the right upper quadrant, and the head is in the left upper quadrant, attached to the duodenum.

The tail of the pancreas touches the spleen. The pancreas releases insulin and glycogen into the bloodstream and produces pancreatic enzymes released into the duodenum for digestion.

Visualize the vascular structures

The abdominal aorta supplies blood to the GI tract. It enters the abdomen, separates into the common iliac arteries, and then branches into many arteries extending the length of the GI tract.

The gastric and splenic veins drain absorbed nutrients into the portal vein of the liver. After entering the liver, the venous blood circulates and then exits the liver through the hepatic vein, emptying into the inferior vena cava.

Obtaining a health history

If your patient has a GI problem, he'll usually complain about pain, heartburn, nausea, vomiting, or altered bowel habits. To investigate these and other chief complaints, ask him about each symptom's onset, duration, and severity.

Knowing what precipitates and relieves the patient's symptoms will help you perform a more accurate physical assessment and better plan your care. (See *Assessing abdominal pain.*)

Asking about past health

To determine whether your patient's problem is new or recurring, ask about past GI illnesses, such as an ulcer, gallbladder disease, inflammatory bowel disease, or GI bleeding. Also ask if he has had abdominal surgery or trauma.

If the patient's chief complaint is diarrhea, find out if he recently traveled abroad. Diarrhea, hepatitis, and parasitic infections can result from ingesting contaminated food or water.

Asking about current health

Ask the patient if he is currently taking medications. Several drugs, including aspirin, sulfonamides, and some antihypertensives, can cause nausea, vomiting, diarrhea, constipation, and other GI symptoms. Be sure to ask about laxative use; habitual use may cause constipation. Also ask

What does it all mean?

Assessing abdominal pain

If your patient complains of abdominal pain, ask him to describe the pain and when and how it started. The table below will help you assess the pain and determine possible causes.

Type of pain	Possible cause
Burning	Peptic ulcer
Cramping	Biliary colic
Severe cramping	Appendicitis
Stabbing	Pancreatitis

Onset of pain	Possible cause
Gradual	Infection
Acute; awakens patient	Duodenal ulcer
Loss of consciousness	Acute pancreatitis, perforated ulcer, ruptured ectopic pregnancy, intestinal obstruction

the patient if he is allergic to medications or foods. Such allergies often cause GI symptoms.

In addition, ask the patient about changes in appetite, difficulty eating or chewing, and changes in bowel habits. Has he noticed a change in the color, amount, and appearance of his stool? Has he ever seen blood in his stool?

Asking about family health

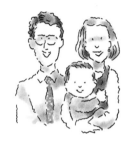

Because some GI disorders are hereditary, ask the patient whether anyone in his family has had a GI disorder. (See *Culture and the GI history.*) Disorders with a familial link include:
- ulcerative colitis
- colon cancer
- stomach ulcers
- diabetes
- alcoholism.
- Crohn's disease.

Asking about psychosocial health

Inquire about your patient's occupation, home life, financial situation, stress level, and recent life changes. Be sure to ask about alcohol, caffeine, and tobacco use as well as food consumption, exercise habits, and oral hygiene. Also ask about sleep patterns: How many hours of sleep does he feel he needs? How many does he get?

Bridging the gap

Culture and the GI history

When taking a health history, consider your patient's ethnic background. For instance, Japanese people are at higher risk than non-Japanese people for gastric cancer, and Native American populations tend to show increased incidences of cirrhosis due to high alcohol consumption.

Assessing the GI system

A physical assessment of the GI system should include a thorough examination of the mouth, abdomen, and rectum. To perform an abdominal assessment, use this sequence: inspection, auscultation, percussion, and palpation. *Palpating or percussing the abdomen before you auscultate can change the character of the patient's bowel sounds and lead to an inaccurate assessment.*

Before beginning your examination, explain what techniques you'll be using, and warn the patient that some procedures might be uncomfortable. Perform the examination in a private, quiet, warm, and well-lighted room.

Examining the mouth

Use inspection and palpation to assess the mouth.

Open wide

First, inspect the patient's mouth and jaw for asymmetry and swelling. Check his bite, noting malocclusion from an overbite or underbite. Inspect the inner and outer lips, teeth, and gums with a pen light. Note bleeding, gum ulcerations, and missing, displaced, or broken teeth. Palpate the gums for tenderness and the inner lips and cheeks for lesions.

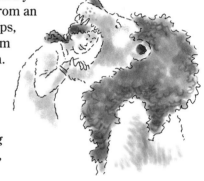

Assess the tongue, checking for coating, tremors, swelling, and ulcerations. Note unusual breath odors. Finally, examine the pharynx, looking for uvular deviation, tonsillar abnormalities, lesions, plaques, and exudate.

Examining the abdomen

Use inspection, auscultation, percussion, and palpation to examine the abdomen. To ensure an accurate assessment, take these actions before the examination:
- Ask the patient to empty his bladder.
- Drape the genitalia and the breasts of a female patient.
- Place a small pillow under the patient's knees to help relax the abdominal muscles.
- Keep the room warm. Chilling can cause abdominal muscles to become tense.
- Keep your fingernails short, and warm your hands and the stethoscope.
- Speak softly, and encourage the patient to perform breathing exercises or use imagery during uncomfortable procedures.
- Assess painful areas last to help prevent the patient from becoming tense.

Inspection

Begin by mentally dividing the abdomen into four quadrants and then imagining the organs in each quadrant. (See *Abdominal quadrants.*)

It's all in the terms

You can more accurately pinpoint your physical findings by knowing these three terms:
- epigastric — above the umbilicus and between the costal margins
- umbilical — around the navel
- suprapubic — above the symphysis pubis.

Checking for a bulge

Observe the abdomen for symmetry, checking for bumps, bulges, or masses. A bulge may indicate bladder distension or hernia.

Abdominal quadrants

To perform a systematic GI assessment, try to visualize the abdominal structures by dividing the abdomen into four quadrants, as shown below.

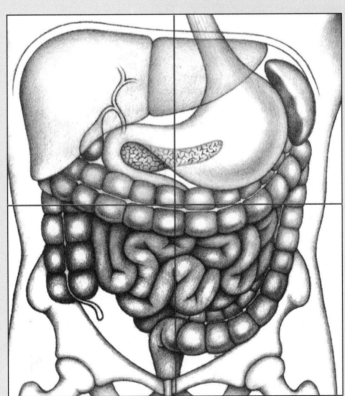

Right upper quadrant
- Right lobe of liver
- Gallbladder
- Pylorus
- Duodenum
- Head of the pancreas
- Hepatic flexure of the colon
- Portions of the ascending and transverse colon

Left upper quadrant
- Left lobe of the liver
- Stomach
- Body of the pancreas
- Splenic flexure of the colon
- Portions of the transverse and descending colon

Right lower quadrant
- Cecum and appendix
- Portion of the ascending colon

Left lower quadrant
- Sigmoid colon
- Portion of the descending colon

Also note the patient's abdominal shape and contour. The abdomen should be flat to rounded in people of average weight. A protruding abdomen may be caused by obesity, pregnancy, ascites, or abdominal distension. A slender person may have a slightly concave abdomen.

Innie or outie?

Assess the umbilicus, which should be located midline in the abdomen and inverted. Conditions such as pregnancy, ascites, or an underlying mass can cause the umbilicus to protrude. Have the patient raise his head and shoulders. If his umbilicus protrudes, he may have an umbilical hernia.

Scouring the skin

The skin of the abdomen should be smooth and uniform in color. Striae, or stretch marks, can be caused by pregnancy, excessive weight gain, or ascites. New striae are pink or blue; old striae are silvery white. Note dilated veins. Record the length of any surgical scars on the abdomen.

Riding the peristaltic wave

Note abdominal movements and pulsations. Usually, waves of peristalsis can't be seen; if they're visible, they look like slight, wavelike motions. Visible rippling waves may indicate bowel obstruction and should be reported immediately. In thin patients, pulsation of the aorta is visible in the epigastric area. Marked pulsations may occur with hypertension, aortic insufficiency, and other conditions causing widening pulse pressure.

Auscultation

Lightly place the stethoscope diaphragm in the right lower quadrant, slightly below and to the right of the umbilicus. Auscultate in a clockwise fashion in each of the four quadrants, spending at least 2 minutes in each area. Note the character and quality of bowel sounds in each quadrant. In some cases, you may need to auscultate for 5 minutes before you hear sounds. Be sure to allow enough time for listening in each quadrant before you decide that bowel sounds are absent.

Before auscultating the abdomen of a patient with a nasogastric tube or another abdominal tube connected to suction, briefly clamp the tube or turn off the suction. Suction noises can obscure or mimic actual bowel sounds.

What does it all mean?

Interpreting abnormal abdominal sounds

Sound and description	Location	Possible cause
Abnormal bowel sounds		
Hyperactive sounds (unrelated to hunger)	Any quadrant	Diarrhea, laxative use, or early intestinal obstruction
Hypoactive, then absent sounds	Any quadrant	Paralytic ileus or peritonitis
High-pitched tinkling sounds	Any quadrant	Intestinal fluid and air under tension in a dilated bowel
High-pitched rushing sounds coinciding with abdominal cramps	Any quadrant	Intestinal obstruction
Systolic bruits		
Vascular blowing sounds resembling cardiac murmurs	Over abdominal aorta	Partial arterial obstruction or turbulent blood flow
	Over renal artery	Renal artery stenosis
	Over iliac artery	Hepatomegaly
Venous hum		
Continuous, medium-pitched tone created by blood flow in a large engorged vascular organ such as the liver	Epigastric and umbilical regions	Increased collateral circulation between portal and systemic venous systems, as in cirrhosis
Friction rub		
Harsh, grating sound like two pieces of sandpaper rubbing together	Over liver and spleen	Inflammation of the peritoneal surface of liver, as from a tumor

Pardon my borborygmus

Normal bowel sounds are high-pitched, gurgling noises caused by air mixing with fluid during peristalsis. The noises vary in frequency, pitch, and intensity and occur irregularly from 5 to 34 times per minute. They're loudest before mealtimes. Borborygmus, or stomach growling, is the loud, gurgling, splashing bowel sound heard over the large intestine as gas passes through it.

Too much activity or not enough?

Bowel sounds are classified as normal, hypoactive, or hyperactive. (See *Interpreting abnormal abdominal sounds,* page 207.) Hyperactive bowel sounds—loud, high-pitched, tinkling sounds that occur frequently—may be caused by diarrhea, constipation, and laxative use.

Hypoactive bowel sounds are heard infrequently. They're associated with ileus, bowel obstruction, or peritonitis and indicate diminished peristalsis. Paralytic ileus, torsion of the bowel, and the use of narcotics and other medications can decrease peristalsis.

Voice of the vessels

Auscultate for vascular sounds with the bell of the stethoscope. (See *Vascular sounds.*) Using firm pressure, listen over the aorta and renal, iliac, and femoral arteries for bruits, venous hums, and friction rubs.

Percussion

Direct or indirect percussion is used to detect the size and location of abdominal organs and to detect air or fluid in the abdomen, stomach, or bowel.

In direct percussion, your hand or finger strikes directly against the patient's abdomen. With indirect percussion, you use the middle finger of your dominant hand or a percussion hammer to strike a finger resting on the patient's abdomen. Begin percussion in the right lower quadrant and proceed clockwise, covering all four quadrants.

Don't percuss the abdomen in a patient with an abdominal aortic aneurysm or a transplanted abdominal organ. It can precipitate a rupture or organ rejection.

Hollow or dull?

You normally hear two sounds during percussion of the abdomen: tympany and dullness. When you percuss over hollow organs, such as an empty stomach or bowel, you hear a clear, hollow sound like a drum beating. This sound, tympany, predominates because air is normally present in the stomach and bowel. The degree of tympany depends on the amount of air and gastric dilation.

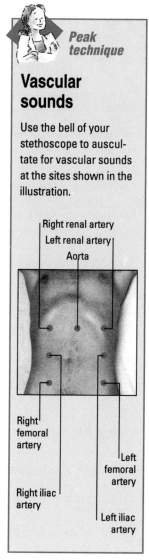

Peak technique

Vascular sounds

Use the bell of your stethoscope to auscultate for vascular sounds at the sites shown in the illustration.

Right renal artery
Left renal artery
Aorta

Right femoral artery

Left femoral artery

Right iliac artery

Left iliac artery

When you percuss over solid organs, such as the liver, kidney, or feces-filled intestines, the sound changes to dullness. Note where percussed sounds change from tympany to dullness. (See *Sites of tympany and dullness*.)

How large is the liver?

Percussion of the liver can help you estimate its size. (See *Percussing and measuring the liver*.) Hepatomegaly is often associated with hepatitis and other liver diseases. Liver borders may be obscured and difficult to assess.

Splenic dullard

The spleen is located at about the level of the 10th rib in the left midaxillary line. Percussion may produce a small area of dullness, generally 7″ (18 cm) or less in adults. However, the spleen usually can't be percussed because tympany from the colon masks the dullness of the spleen.

Conditions that cause splenomegaly include mononucleosis, trauma, and illnesses that destroy red blood cells, such as sickle cell anemia and some cancers. (See *Spleen or kidney enlargement?* page 210.) To assess for splenic enlargement, ask the patient to breathe deeply. Then percuss along the 9th to 11th intercostal spaces on the left,

Sites of tympany and dullness

Expect to auscultate tympany and dullness in the areas shown here.

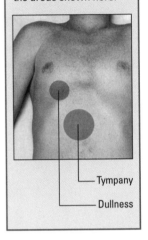

Tympany

Dullness

Peak technique

Percussing and measuring the liver

To percuss and measure the liver, follow these steps:
• Identify the upper border of liver dullness. Start in the right midclavicular line in an area of lung resonance, and then percuss downward toward the liver. Use a pen to mark the spot where the sound changes to dullness.
• Start in the right midclavicular line at a level below the umbilicus, and lightly percuss upward toward the liver. Mark the spot where the sound changes from tympany to dullness.
• Use a ruler to measure the vertical span between the two marked spots, as shown. In an adult, a normal liver span ranges from 2 ½″ to 4 ¾″ (6.5 to 12 cm).

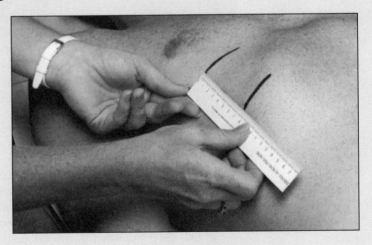

listening for a change from tympany to dullness. Measure the area of dullness.

Palpation

Abdominal palpation includes light and deep touch to help determine the size, shape, position, and tenderness of major abdominal organs, and to detect masses and fluid accumulation. Palpate all four quadrants, leaving painful and tender areas for last. (See *Recognizing types of abdominal pain.*)

Light touch

Light palpation helps identify muscle resistance and tenderness as well as the location of some superficial organs. To palpate, put the fingers of one hand close together, depress the skin about ½″ (1.3 cm) with your fingertips, and make gentle, rotating movements. Avoid short, quick jabs.

The abdomen should be soft and nontender. As you palpate the four quadrants, note organs, masses, and areas of tenderness or increased resistance. Determine whether resistance is due to the patient's being cold, tense, or ticklish or whether it's from involuntary guarding or rigidity from muscle spasms or peritoneal inflammation.

Help the ticklish patient relax by putting his hand over yours as you palpate. If he complains of abdominal tenderness even before you touch him, palpate by placing your stethoscope lightly on his abdomen.

Deep palpation

To perform deep palpation, push the abdomen down about 2″ to 3″ (5 to 7.5 cm). In an obese patient, put one hand on top of the other and push. Palpate the entire abdomen in a clockwise direction, checking for tenderness, pulsations, organ enlargement, and masses.

If the patient's abdomen is rigid, don't palpate it. He could have peritoneal inflammation, and palpation could cause pain or rupture an inflamed organ.

Palpating the liver and spleen

Palpate the patient's liver to check for enlargement and tenderness. (See *Palpating the liver,* page 212.) Unless the spleen is enlarged, it isn't palpable. *If you do feel the spleen, stop palpating immediately because compression can cause rupture.* (See *Palpating the spleen,* page 213.)

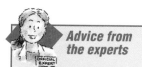

Advice from the experts

Spleen or kidney enlargement?

To differentiate between spleen and kidney enlargement, ask your patient to take a deep breath. Then percuss along the 9th and 10th intercostal spaces. You should hear tympany produced by colonic or gastric air. If you hear dullness instead, the patient's spleen may be enlarged. If you hear resonance, his left kidney may be enlarged.

What does it all mean?

Recognizing types of abdominal pain

What can you do to figure out which organ is affected if your patient has abdominal pain? Assess the location of his pain and then look at this chart to get a quick idea of the most likely source of the pain.

Affected organ	Visceral pain	Parietal pain	Referred pain
Stomach	Midepigastrium	Midepigastrium and left upper quadrant	Shoulders
Small intestine	Periumbilical area	Over affected site	Midback (rare)
Appendix	Periumbilical area	Right lower quadrant	Right lower quadrant
Proximal colon	Periumbilical area and right flank for ascending colon	Over affected site	Right lower quadrant and back (rare)
Distal colon	Hypogastrium and left flank for descending colon	Over affected site	Left lower quadrant and back (rare)
Gallbladder	Midepigastrium	Right upper quadrant	Right subscapular area
Ureters	Costovertebral angle	Over affected site	Groin; scrotum in men, labia in women (rare)
Pancreas	Midepigastrium and left upper quadrant	Midepigastrium and left upper quadrant	Back and left shoulder
Ovaries, fallopian tubes, and uterus	Hypogastrium and groin	Over affected site	Inner thighs

Special assessment procedures

To check for rebound tenderness or ascites, use the following procedures.

On the rebound

Perform the test for rebound tenderness when you suspect peritoneal inflammation. Check for rebound at the end of your examination.

Choosing a site away from the painful area, position your hand at a 90-degree angle to the abdomen. Push down slowly and deeply into the abdomen, and then withdraw your hand quickly. Rapid withdrawal causes the underlying structures to rebound suddenly and results in a sharp, stabbing pain on the inflamed side. *Don't repeat this maneuver or you may rupture an inflamed appendix.*

Fluid overload

Ascites, a large accumulation of fluid in the peritoneal cavity, can be caused by advanced liver disease, heart failure, pancreatitis, or cancer.

Peak technique

Palpating the liver

These illustrations show the correct hand positions for two ways of palpating the liver.

Palpating the liver
• Place the patient in the supine position. Standing at his right side, place your left hand under his back at the approximate location of the liver.
• Place your right hand slightly below the mark you made earlier at the liver's upper border. Point the fingers of your right hand toward the patient's head just under the right costal margin.
• As the patient inhales deeply, gently press in and up on the abdomen until the liver brushes under your right hand. The edge should be smooth, firm, and somewhat round. Note tenderness.

Hooking the liver
• Hooking is an alternate way of palpating the liver. To hook the liver, stand next to the patient's right shoulder, facing his feet. Place your hands side by side, and hook your fingertips over the right costal margin, below the lower mark of dullness.
• Ask the patient to take a deep breath as you push your fingertips in and up. If the liver is palpable, you may feel its edge as it slides down in the abdomen with inspiration.

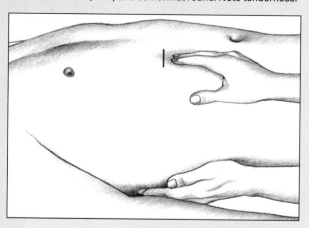

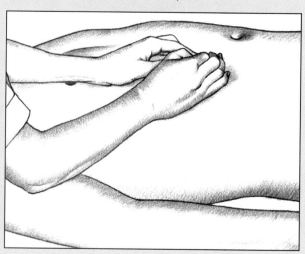

If ascites is present, use a tape measure to measure the fullest part of the abdomen. Mark this point on the patient's abdomen with indelible ink so you'll be sure to measure it consistently. This measurement is important, especially if fluid removal or paracentesis is performed. (See *Checking for ascites*, page 214.)

Examining the rectum and anus

If your patient is age 40 or over, perform a rectal examination as part of your GI assessment. Be sure to explain the procedure to the patient.

Inspect the outside

First, inspect the perianal area. Put on gloves and spread the buttocks to expose the anus and surrounding tissue, checking for fissures, lesions, scars, inflammation, discharge, rectal prolapse, and external hemorrhoids. Asking the patient to strain as if he's having a bowel movement may reveal internal hemorrhoids, polyps, or fissures. The skin in the perianal area is normally somewhat darker than that of the surrounding area.

Palpate the inside

Next palpate the rectum. Apply a water-soluble lubricant to your gloved index finger. Tell the patient to relax, and warn him that he'll feel some pressure. Then insert your finger into the rectum, toward the umbilicus. To palpate as much of the rectal wall as possible, rotate your finger clockwise, then counterclockwise. The rectal walls should feel soft and smooth, without masses, fecal impaction, or tenderness.

Inspect and test

Remove your finger from the rectum, and inspect the glove for stool, blood, and mucus. Test fecal matter adhering to the glove for occult blood using a guaiac test.

Abnormal findings

GI disorders can affect a patient's ingestion, digestion, and elimination. This section describes common abnormalities you might uncover during a GI assessment.

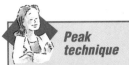

Peak technique

Palpating the spleen

Although a normal spleen isn't palpable, an enlarged spleen is. To palpate the spleen, stand on the patient's right side. Use your left hand to support his posterior left lower rib cage. Ask him to take a deep breath. Then, with your right hand on his abdomen, press up and in toward the spleen.

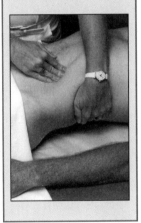

Nausea and vomiting

Usually occurring together, nausea and vomiting can be caused by existing illnesses, such as myocardial infarction, gastric and peritoneal irritation, appendicitis, bowel obstruction, cholecystitis, acute pancreatitis, and neurologic disturbances.

Dysphagia

Dysphagia, or difficulty in talking, eating, or swallowing, may be accompanied by weight loss. It can be caused by an obstruction, achalasia of the lower esophagogastric junction, or a neurologic disease, such as stroke or impaired motor activity. Dysphagia can lead to aspiration.

Skin color changes

A bluish umbilicus, called Cullen's sign, indicates intra-abdominal hemorrhage. Areas of abdominal redness may indicate inflammation. Bruising on the flank, or Turner's sign, indicates retroperitoneal hemorrhage. Dilated, tortuous, visible abdominal veins may indicate inferior vena cava obstruction. Cutaneous angiomas may signal liver disease.

Constipation

Constipation can be caused by immobility, a sedentary lifestyle, or medications. The patient may complain of a dull ache in the abdomen, a full feeling, and hyperactive bowel sounds, which may be caused by irritable bowel syndrome. A patient with complete intestinal obstruction won't pass flatus or stool and won't have bowel sounds below the obstruction. Constipation occurs more commonly in older patients.

Diarrhea

Diarrhea may be caused by toxins, medications, or a GI disease such as Crohn's disease. Cramping, abdominal tenderness, anorexia, and hyperactive bowel sounds may accompany diarrhea. If fever occurs, the diarrhea may be caused by a toxin.

Abdominal distension

Distension may occur with gas, a tumor, or a colon filled with feces. It may also be caused by an incisional hernia, which may protrude when the patient lifts his head and shoulders.

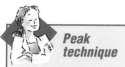

Peak technique

Checking for ascites

To check for ascites, have an assistant place the ulnar edge of her hand firmly on the patient's abdomen at its midline. Then, as you stand facing the patient's head, place the palm of your right hand against the patient's left flank. Give the right abdomen a firm tap with your left hand, as shown. If ascites is present, you may see and feel a "fluid wave" ripple across the abdomen.

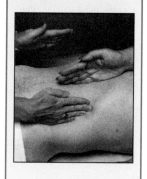

Abnormal bowel sounds

Hyperactive bowel sounds indicate increased intestinal motility and have many causes, including laxative use, gastroenteritis, and life-threatening intestinal obstruction. Hypoactive bowel sounds can be caused by recent bowel surgery, a full colon, or paralytic ileus.

Friction rubs

Friction rubs over the liver and spleen in the epigastric region may indicate splenic infarction or hepatic tumor. Abdominal bruits may be caused by aortic aneurysms or partial arterial obstruction.

Abdominal pain

Abdominal pain may result from ulcers, intestinal obstruction, appendicitis, cholecystitis, peritonitis, or other inflammatory disorders. A duodenal ulcer can cause gnawing abdominal pain in the midepigastrium 2 to 4 hours after eating. The pain may awaken the patient and be relieved by antacids or food.

Rebound tenderness can be caused by peritonitis or appendicitis. Appendicitis may be accompanied by increased abdominal wall resistance and guarding. Not all patients have the classic right lower quadrant pain. Some older adults with appendicitis have less abdominal rigidity than younger patients.

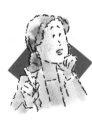

Quick quiz

1. When food is swallowed, the epiglottis:
   A. opens.
   B. closes.
   C. opens or closes, depending on the type of food.

Answer: B. The epiglottis, a thin flap of tissue over the larynx, closes during swallowing to prevent aspiration.

2. The correct sequence for an abdominal assessment is:
   A. inspection, percussion, palpation, and auscultation.
   B. percussion, auscultation, inspection, and palpation.
   C. inspection, auscultation, percussion, and palpation.

Answer: C. Percussion and palpation can increase intestinal motility and bowel sounds, so inspection and auscultation must be done first.

3. Hyperactive bowel sounds may be a sign of:
    A. ileus or bowel obstruction.
    B. peritonitis or narcotic use.
    C. constipation, diarrhea, or laxative use.

Answer: C. Hyperactive bowel sounds are a sign of constipation, diarrhea, or laxative use.

4. When you percuss over the liver, you should hear:
    A. dullness.
    B. resonance.
    C. tympany.

Answer: A. Percussing over solid organs, such as the liver or kidney, should create a dull sound.

5. If you suspect splenomegaly during abdominal palpation, you should:
    A. continue to palpate.
    B. stop palpation immediately.
    C. palpate more gently, working your way laterally from the midline of the abdomen.

Answer: B. The spleen isn't palpable unless it's enlarged. If you suspect splenomegaly, stop palpation because it can cause the spleen to rupture.

6. To test a patient for rebound tenderness, position your hand at a:
    A. 30-degree angle to the abdomen.
    B. 45- to 60-degree angle to the abdomen.
    C. 90-degree angle to the abdomen.

Answer: C. Choosing a site away from the painful area, position your hand at a 90-degree angle to the abdomen. Push down slowly and deeply into the abdomen, and then withdraw your hand quickly.

Scoring

★★★   If you answered all six items correctly, congratulations! You win a trip to the Island of Borborygmus!

★★   If you answered four or five correctly, super! You win a trip to the Grand Tympany Resort!

★   If you answered fewer than four items correctly, alright! You win a trip down the breathtaking Alimentary Canal, with your captain, Perry Stalsis!

11

Female genitourinary system

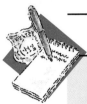

Just the facts

This chapter discusses the female genitourinary (GU) system and how to assess it. In this chapter, you'll learn:

♦ what organs and structures make up the female GU system

♦ how to obtain a patient history

♦ how to perform a physical assessment of the female GU system

♦ how to recognize female GU system abnormalities.

A look at the female GU system

The female GU system encompasses the urinary tract and the reproductive organs and structures. Disorders of this system can have wide-ranging effects on other body systems. For example, ovarian dysfunction can alter endocrine balance, and kidney dysfunction can affect the production of the hormone erythropoietin, which regulates the production of red blood cells.

Assessing the female GU system can be a challenging task. Many patients with urinary disorders don't realize they're ill because they have only mild signs and symptoms. So it's easy to overlook underlying problems.

In addition, more women seek health care for reproductive disorders than for anything else. Assessing those problems can be difficult because the reproductive system is complex and its functions have far-reaching psychosocial implications.

Urinary system

The urinary system consists of the kidneys, ureters, bladder, and urethra. (See *Urinary system*.) Let's look at each one in turn.

Kidneys

The essential functions of the urinary system — such as forming urine and maintaining homeostasis — take place in the highly vascular kidneys. These bean-shaped organs are 4½″ to 5″ (11.5 to 12.5 cm) long and 2½″ (6.5 cm) wide. Located retroperitoneally on either side of the lumbar vertebrae, the kidneys lie behind the abdominal organs and in front of the muscles attached to the vertebral column. The peritoneal fat layer protects them.

Urinary system

The illustration below shows the main structures of the urinary system.

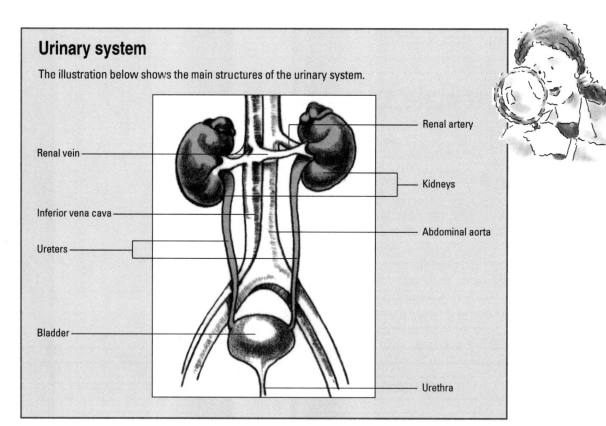

Renal vein

Inferior vena cava

Ureters

Bladder

Renal artery

Kidneys

Abdominal aorta

Urethra

Makin' urine

Crowded by the liver, the right kidney extends slightly lower than the left. Each kidney contains roughly one million nephrons. Urine gathers in collecting tubules and ducts and eventually drains into the ureters, down into the bladder and, when urination occurs, out through the urethra.

Ureters

The ureters are about 10″ to 12″ (25.5 to 30.5 cm) long. The left ureter is slightly longer than the right because of the left kidney's higher position. The diameter of each ureter varies from ⅛″ to ¼″ (3 to 6 mm), with the narrowest part at the ureteropelvic junction.

The rhythm of the flow

Located along the posterior abdominal wall, the ureters enter the bladder anteromedially. They carry urine from the kidneys to the bladder by peristaltic contractions that occur one to five times per minute.

Bladder

Located in the pelvis, the bladder is a container for urine collection. Bladder capacity ranges from 500 to 1,000 ml in healthy adults, less in children and elderly people. When the bladder is empty, it lies behind the pelvic bone; when it's full, it becomes displaced under the peritoneal cavity.

Urethra

A small duct, the urethra carries urine from the bladder to the outside of the body. A woman's urethra is only 1″ to 2″ (2.5 to 5 cm) long and opens anterior to the vaginal opening.

Reproductive system

The female reproductive system consists of external and internal genitalia. Let's start with external genitalia.

External genitalia

The external genitalia, collectively called the vulva, consist of the mons pubis, labia majora, labia minora, clitoris, vagina, urethra, and Skene's and Bartholin's glands. (See *External genitalia*.)

Mons pubis

The mons pubis is a mound of adipose tissue overlying the symphysis pubis and is covered with pubic hair in the adult. Pubic hair first appears on average at age 10½. It may become sparse after menopause due to hormonal changes. Native Americans and Asians usually have less pubic hair than people of other races.

Labia majora and minora

The outer vulval lips, or labia majora, are two rounded folds of adipose tissue that extend from the mons pubis to the perineum. The labia majora is covered with hair.

The inner vulval lips are called the labia minora. The anterolateral and medial parts join to form the prepuce and frenulum, the folds of skin that cap the clitoris. The posterior union of the labia minora is called the fourchette.

External genitalia

The illustration below shows the main parts of the external female genitalia.

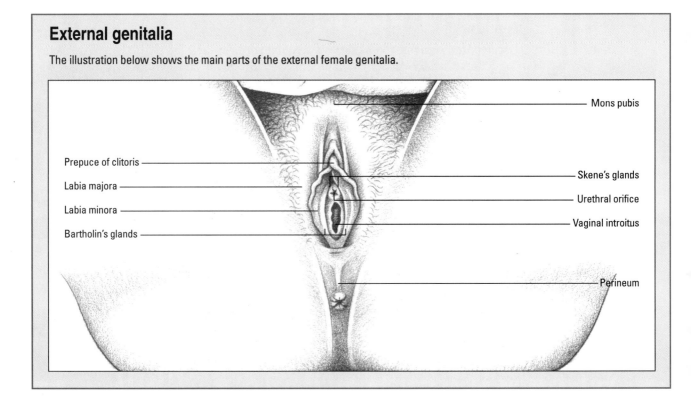

Clitoris, vestibule, and urethral opening

The clitoris is composed of erectile tissue and lies between the labia minora at the top of the vestibule, which contains the urethral and vaginal openings. The urethral opening is a slit below the clitoris.

Vaginal opening and perineum

The vaginal opening, or introitus, is posterior to the urethral orifice. This opening is a thin vertical slit in women with intact hymens and a large opening with irregular edges in women whose hymens have been perforated. In some women, the hymen is absent.

The perineum is the area bordered anteriorly by the top of the labial fold and posteriorly by the anus.

Skene's and Bartholin's glands

Two kinds of glands have ducts that open into the vulva. Skene's glands are tiny structures just below the urethra, each containing 6 to 31 ducts. Bartholin's glands are found posterior to the vaginal opening. Neither of these glands can be seen, but they can be palpated if enlarged.

Skene's and Bartholin's glands produce fluids important for the reproductive process. They can become infected, usually with organisms known to cause sexually transmitted diseases (STDs).

Internal genitalia

The internal genitalia include the vagina, uterus, ovaries, and fallopian tubes. (See *Internal genitalia,* page 222.)

Vagina

A pink, hollow, collapsed tube, the vagina is located between the urethra and the rectum, extending up and back from the vulva to the uterus. It is the route of passage for childbirth and menstruation.

Uterus

The uterus is a hollow, pear-shaped, muscular organ that lies between the rectum and the bladder. It's divided into the fundus and the cervix, which protrudes into the vagina. The cervix contains mucus-secreting glands that help in reproduction and protect the uterus from pathogens. The function of the uterus is to nurture and then expel the fetus.

Internal genitalia

The illustration below shows the main internal structures of the female reproductive system.

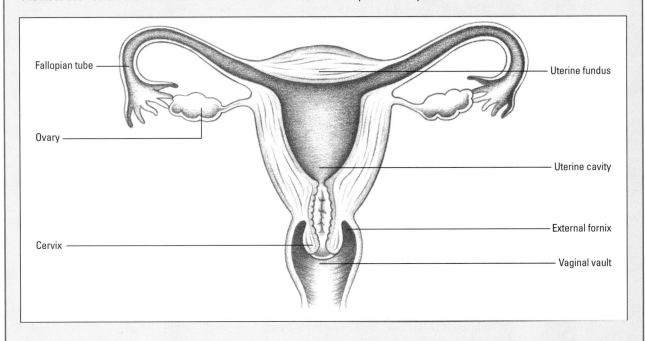

The position of the uterus in the pelvic cavity may vary, depending on bladder fullness. The uterus may also tip in different directions.

Ovaries

A pair of oval organs about 1¼″ (3 cm) long, the ovaries are usually found near the lateral pelvic wall at the height of the anterosuperior iliac spine. They produce ova and release the hormones estrogen and progesterone. The ovaries become fully developed after puberty and shrink after menopause.

Fallopian tubes

Each approximately 4″ (10 cm) long, the two fallopian tubes extend from the ovaries into the upper portion of the uterus. Their funnel-shaped ends curve toward the ovaries and, during ovulation, help guide the ova to the uterus after expulsion from the ovaries. The fallopian tube is also the usual site of fertilization of the ova by the sperm.

Obtaining a health history

Because the urinary and reproductive systems are located so close together in women, you and your patient may have trouble differentiating signs and symptoms. Even if the patient's complaint seems minor, investigate it. Ask about its onset, duration, and severity and about measures taken to treat it. The information you gain will help you formulate a more appropriate plan of care.

Asking about the urinary system

The most common chief complaints of the urinary system include output changes, such as polyuria, oliguria, and anuria; voiding pattern changes, such as hesitancy, frequency, urgency, nocturia, and incontinence; urine color changes; and pain.

Asking about past health

Past illnesses and preexisting conditions can affect a patient's urinary tract health. For example, has the patient ever had a urinary tract infection (UTI), kidney trauma, or kidney stones? Kidney stones or trauma can alter the structure and function of the kidneys and bladder.

Asking about current health

Ask the patient about current problems and medications. Does the patient have diabetes or hypertension? Patients with diabetes have an increased risk of UTIs. Hypertension can contribute to renal failure and nephropathy.

Has she noticed a change in the color or odor of her urine? Does she have problems with incontinence or frequency? Does she have allergies? Allergic reactions can cause tubular damage. A severe anaphylactic reaction can cause temporary renal failure and permanent tubular necrosis.

Make a list of the prescribed medications and over-the-counter drugs the patient takes. Some drugs can affect the appearance of urine; nephrotoxic drugs can alter urinary function. Also ask about the patient's family, to get information about her risk of developing kidney failure or kidney disease.

Asking about the reproductive system

The most common reproductive system complaints are pain, vaginal discharge, abnormal uterine bleeding, pruritus, and infertility. To obtain the most complete data about those problems, focus on the patient's current complaints, and then explore her reproductive, sexual-social, and family history. Ask her to describe symptoms in her own words, encouraging her to speak freely.

Many patients feel uncomfortable answering questions about their sexual health or reproductive system. So start with the less personal questions to establish a rapport.

Asking about menstruation

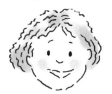

Start by asking about her menstrual cycle. How old was she when she began to menstruate? How long does her period usually last? How often does it occur? The normal cycle for menstruation is one menses every 21 to 38 days. The normal duration is 2 to 8 days.

Does she have cramps, spotting, or an unusually heavy or light flow? Spotting between periods, or metrorrhagia, may be normal in patients taking low-dose oral contraceptives or progesterone; otherwise, spotting may indicate infection or cancer.

In girls, menses generally starts by age 14. If it hasn't, and if no secondary sex characteristics have developed, the patient should be evaluated by a doctor.

Asking about menopause

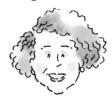

If your patient is postmenopausal, ask for the date of her last menstrual period. Is she having hot flashes, mood swings, or flushing? Also ask these questions of a postmenopausal woman — or any woman: Does she have vaginal discharge, other than a normal, clear, nonodorous discharge? Does she have external lesions or itching? Does she douche, and if so, how often? When was her last Papanicolaou (Pap) smear, and what was the result?

Asking about pregnancy

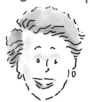

Ask the patient if she has ever been pregnant. If so, how many times has she been pregnant, and how many times did she give birth? Did she have a vaginal delivery or cesarean section? What kind of birth control, if any, does she use? If the patient is sexually active, talk to her about the importance of safe sex and the prevention of STDs.

Asking about sexual practices

Once the patient seems comfortable, ask her about her sexual practices, the number of sexual partners she currently has, whether she has ever had an STD, and her human immunodeficiency virus status. Be sure to ask if she has questions or concerns.

Assessing the female GU system

To perform a physical assessment of the GU system, you'll use the techniques of inspection, percussion, and palpation to evaluate the urinary and reproductive systems. We'll look at the urinary system first.

Examining the urinary system

Before assessing specific structures of the urinary system, evaluate your patient's vital signs, weight, and mental status. These observations will provide clues about renal dysfunction.

For example, a patient's vital signs might reveal hypertension, which can cause renal dysfunction if it's uncontrolled. Be sure to check blood pressure in each arm. Weighing the patient can provide information about fluid status and is important for patients with urinary disorders or renal failure, especially those receiving dialysis.

Observing mental status

Observing the patient's behavior can give you clues about her mental status. Does she have trouble concentrating, have memory loss, or seem disoriented? Kidney dysfunction can cause those symptoms. Progressive, chronic kidney failure can cause lethargy, confusion, disorientation, stupor, convulsions, and coma.

Inspection

First, observe the color and shape of the area around the kidneys and bladder. The skin should be free from lesions, discolorations, and swelling.

Percussion

Kidney percussion checks for costovertebral angle tenderness that occurs with inflammation. To percuss over the kidneys, have the patient sit up. Place the ball of your non-dominant hand on her back at the costovertebral angle of the 12th rib. Strike the ball of that hand with the ulnar surface of your other hand. Use just enough force to cause a painless but perceptible thud.

The bladder matters

To percuss the bladder, first ask the patient to empty it. Then have her lie in the supine position. Start at the symphysis pubis and percuss upward toward the bladder and over it. You should hear tympany. A dull sound signals retained urine.

Palpation

Because the kidneys lie behind other organs and are protected by muscle, they normally aren't palpable unless they're enlarged. (See *Palpating the kidneys*.) However, in very thin patients, you may be able to feel the lower end of the right kidney as a smooth round mass that drops on inspiration.

In elderly patients, you may be able to palpate both kidneys because of decreased muscle tone and elasticity. If the kidneys feel enlarged, the patient may have hydronephrosis, cysts, or tumors.

If the bladder is full, you'll feel it

You won't be able to palpate the bladder unless it's distended. With the patient supine, use the fingers of one hand to palpate the lower abdomen in a light dipping motion. A distended bladder will feel firm and relatively smooth. If the patient is about 12 weeks or more pregnant, you might actually be feeling the fundus of the uterus, palpable just above the symphysis pubis.

Examining the reproductive system

Before the examination, ask the patient to void to prevent discomfort and inaccurate findings during palpation. Have her disrobe and put on an examination gown. Help her into the dorsal lithotomy position, and drape all areas not being examined. Make sure you explain the procedure to her.

You'll begin by examining her external genitalia, and then her internal genitalia.

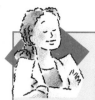

Peak technique

Palpating the kidneys

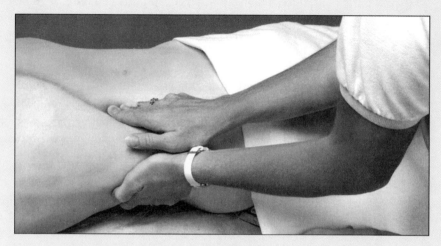

To palpate the kidneys, first have the patient lie supine. To palpate the right kidney, stand on her right side. Then place your left hand under her back and your right hand on her abdomen.

Instruct her to inhale deeply, so her kidney moves downward. As she inhales, press up with your left hand and down with your right, as shown.

Inspecting the external genitalia

First, put on a pair of gloves. Spread the labia and locate the urethral meatus. It should be a pink, irregular, slitlike opening at the midline, just above the vagina. Note the presence of discharge (a sign of urethral infection) or ulcerations (a sign of an STD).

Check the pubic hair

Inspect the external genitalia and pubic hair to assess sexual maturity. Pubic hair changes in density, color, and texture throughout a woman's life. Before adolescence, the pubic area is covered only with body hair. In adolescence, this hair grows thicker, darker, coarser, and curlier. In full maturity, it spreads over the symphysis pubis and inner thighs. In later years, the hair grows thin, gray, and brittle.

Check the labia

Using your index finger and thumb, gently spread the labia majora and minora. They should be moist and free from lesions. You may detect a normal discharge varying from clear and stretchy before ovulation to white and opaque after ovulation. The discharge should be odorless and nonirritating to the mucosa.

Check the vestibule

Examine the vestibule, especially the area around the Bartholin's and Skene's glands. Check for swelling, redness, lesions, discharge, and unusual odor. If you detect any of those conditions, notify the doctor and obtain a specimen for culture. Finally, inspect the vaginal opening, noting whether the hymen is intact or perforated.

Palpating the external genitalia

Spread the labia with one hand and palpate with the other. The labia should feel soft. Note swelling, hardness, or tenderness. If you detect a mass or lesion, palpate it to determine its size, shape, and consistency.

A gentle touch

If you find swelling or tenderness, see if you can palpate Bartholin's glands, which normally aren't palpable. To do this, insert your finger carefully into the patient's posterior introitus, and place your thumb along the lateral edge of the swollen or tender labium. Gently squeeze the labium. If discharge from the duct results, culture it.

Inflamed urethra

If the urethra is inflamed, milk it and the area of Skene's glands. First, moisten your gloved index finger with water. Then separate the labia with your other hand, and insert your index finger about 1¼″ (3 cm) into the anterior vagina. With the pad of your finger, gently press and pull outward. Continue palpating down to the introitus. This procedure shouldn't cause the patient discomfort. Culture the discharge.

Inspecting the internal genitalia

Nurses don't routinely inspect internal genitalia unless they're in advanced practice. However, you may be asked to assist with this examination. To start, select an appropriate speculum for your patient. (See *Speculum types*.)

Getting ready

Hold the speculum under warm, running water to lubricate and warm the blades. Don't use lubricants; many of them are bacteriostatic and can alter results of Pap tests.

Then sit or stand at the foot of the examination table. Tell the patient she'll feel internal pressure and possibly some slight, transient discomfort as you insert and open the speculum.

Relax, insert

Using your dominant hand, hold the speculum by the base, with the blades anchored between your index and middle fingers. (See *Inserting a speculum,* page 230.) This keeps the blades from accidentally opening during insertion. Encourage the patient to take slow, deep breaths during insertion to relax her abdominal muscles.

Speculum types

Specula come in various shapes and sizes. Choose an appropriate one for your patient. A Grave's speculum is usually used. However, if the patient has an intact hymen, has never given birth through the vaginal canal, or has a contracted introitus from menopause, use a Pederson speculum. The illustrations below show the parts of a typical speculum and three types of specula.

Parts of a speculum

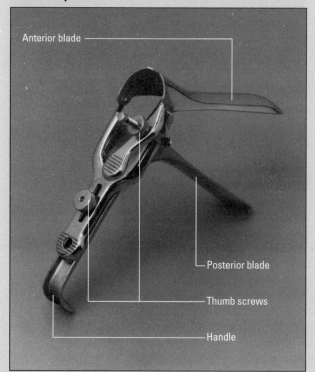

Anterior blade

Posterior blade

Thumb screws

Handle

Types of specula

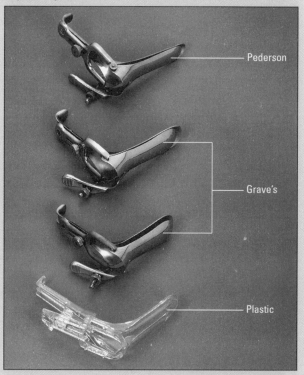

Pederson

Grave's

Plastic

A look inside

After inserting the speculum, observe the color, texture, and integrity of the vaginal lining. A thin, white, odorless discharge on the vaginal walls is normal. Using the thumb of the hand holding the speculum, press the lower lever to open the blades. Then lock them in the open position by tightening the thumb screw above the lever.

Examine the cervix for color, position, size, shape, mucosal integrity, and discharge. It should be smooth and round. The central cervical opening, or cervical os, is circular in a woman who hasn't given birth vaginally and a horizontal slit in a women who has. (See *The normal os.*) Expect to see a clear, watery cervical discharge during

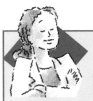

Peak technique

Inserting a speculum

Proper positioning and insertion of the speculum are important for the comfort of the patient and for proper visualization of internal structures. The illustration shows the proper angle and hand position for insertion.

Initial insertion
Place the index and middle fingers of your nondominant hand about 1" (2.5 cm) into the vagina and spread the fingers to exert pressure on the posterior vagina. Hold the speculum in your dominant hand, and insert the blades between your fingers as shown.

Deeper insertion
Ask the patient to bear down to open the introitus and relax the perineal muscles. Point the speculum slightly downward, and insert the blades until the base of the speculum touches your fingers, inside the vagina.

Rotate and open
Then rotate the speculum in the same plane as the vagina, and withdraw your fingers. Open the blades as far as possible and lock them. You should now be able to view the cervix clearly.

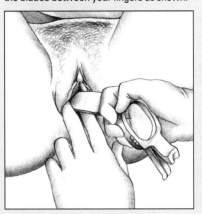
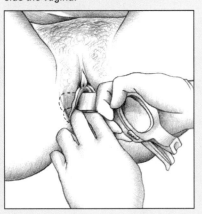
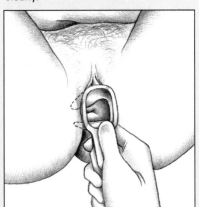

ovulation and a slightly bloody discharge just before menstruation.

Use the speculum to obtain a specimen for a Pap test. Finally, unlock and close the blades and withdraw the speculum.

Palpating the internal genitalia

To palpate the internal genitalia, lubricate the index and middle fingers of your gloved dominant hand. Stand at the foot of the examination table and position this hand for insertion into the vagina by extending your thumb, index, and middle fingers and curling your ring and little finger toward your palm.

Use the thumb and index finger of your other hand to spread the labia majora. Insert your two lubricated fingers into the vagina, exerting pressure posteriorly to avoid irritating the anterior wall and urethra.

Check the vaginal wall and urethra

When your fingers are fully inserted, note tenderness or nodularity in the vaginal wall. Ask the patient to bear down so you can assess the support of the vaginal outlet. Bulging of the vaginal wall may indicate a cystocele or a rectocele.

Check the cervix

To palpate the cervix, sweep your fingers from side to side across the cervix and around the os. The cervix should be smooth and firm and protrude ½″ to 1¼″ (1.3 to 3 cm) into the vagina. If you palpate nodules or irregularities, the patient may have cysts, tumors, or other lesions.

Next place your fingers into the recessed area around the cervix. The cervix should move in all directions. If the patient reports pain during this part of the examination, she may have uterine or inflammation of the adnexa (ovaries, uterine tubes, and ligaments of the uterus).

Bimanual palpation

A bimanual examination allows you to palpate the uterus and ovaries. (See *Performing a bimanual examination,* page 232.) Usually, only nurses in advanced practice perform bimanual palpation.

The normal os

These illustrations show the difference between the os of a woman who has never given birth vaginally (nulliparous) and the os of a woman who has (parous).

Nulliparous

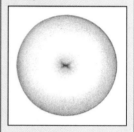

Parous

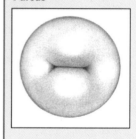

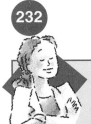

Peak technique

Performing a bimanual examination

During a bimanual examination, you palpate the uterus and ovaries from the inside and the outside simultaneously. The illustrations below show how to perform such an examination.

Proper position

After donning gloves, place the index and third fingers of your dominant hand in the patient's vagina and move them up to the cervix. Place the fingers of your other hand on the patient's abdomen between the umbilicus and the symphysis pubis, as shown.

Elevate the cervix and uterus by pressing upward with the two fingers inside the vagina. At the same time, press down and in with the hand on the abdomen. Try to grasp the uterus between your hands.

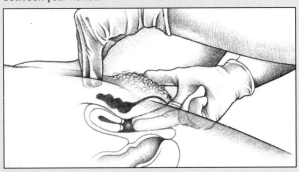

Palpate the walls

Slide your fingers farther into the anterior section of the fornix, the space between the uterus and cervix. You should feel part of the posterior uterine wall with this hand. You should feel part of the anterior uterine wall with the fingertips of your nondominant hand. Note the size, shape, surface characteristics, consistency, and mobility of the uterus as well as tenderness.

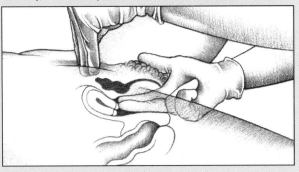

Note the position

Now move your fingers into the posterior fornix, pressing upward and forward to bring the anterior uterine wall up to your nondominant hand. Use your dominant hand to palpate the lower portion of the uterine wall. Note the position of the uterus.

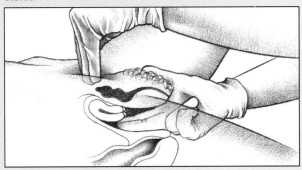

Palpate the ovaries

After palpating the anterior and posterior walls of the uterus, move your nondominant hand toward the right lower quadrant of the abdomen. Slip the fingers of your dominant hand into the right fornix and palpate the right ovary. Then palpate the left ovary. Note the size, shape, and contour of each ovary. They should be unpalpable in postmenopausal women. Remove your hand from the patient's abdomen and your fingers from her vagina, and discard your gloves.

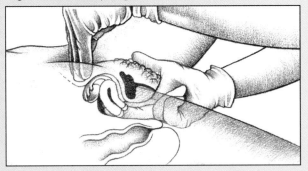

Rectovaginal palpation

Rectovaginal palpation, the last step in a genital assessment, examines the posterior part of the uterus and the pelvic cavity. Warn the patient that this procedure may be uncomfortable.

Put a new pair of gloves on and apply water-soluble lubricant to the index and middle fingers of your gloved dominant hand. Instruct the patient to bear down with her vaginal and rectal muscles; then insert your index finger a short way into her vagina and your middle finger into her rectum.

Palpating the rectum

Use your middle finger to assess rectal muscle and sphincter tone. Insert your finger deeper into the rectum, and palpate the rectal wall with your middle finger. Sweep the rectum with your fingers, assessing for masses or nodules.

Palpate the posterior wall of the uterus through the anterior wall of the rectum, evaluating the uterus for size, shape, tenderness, and masses. The rectovaginal septum, the wall between the rectum and the vagina, should feel smooth and springy.

Feeling the edges

Place your nondominant hand on the patient's abdomen at the symphysis pubis. With your index finger in the vagina, palpate deeply to feel the posterior edge of the cervix and the lower posterior wall of the uterus.

When you're finished, discard the gloves and wash your hands. Help the patient to a sitting position, and provide privacy for dressing and personal hygiene.

Abnormal findings

In addition to the disorders already discussed, your assessment may uncover other abnormalities of the GU system. We'll start with abnormalities in the urinary system.

Urinary abnormalities

Common abnormal findings in the female urinary system include polyuria; hematuria; urinary frequency, urgency, and hesitancy; nocturia; urinary incontinence; and dysuria.

Polyuria

A fairly common finding, polyuria is the production and excretion of more than 2,500 ml of urine daily. It usually results from diabetes insipidus, diabetes mellitus, or diuretic use.

Plenty of causes of polyuria

Other causes of polyuria include psychological, neurologic, or renal disorders. Urologic disorders, such as pyelonephritis and postobstructive uropathy, can also cause polyuria. Patients with polyuria are at risk for developing hypovolemia.

Hematuria

Hematuria causes brown or bright red urine. The timing of hematuria suggests the location of the underlying problem. Bleeding at the start of urination is caused by a disorder of the urethra; bleeding at the end of urination signifies a disorder of the bladder neck.

Above or below the neck

When bleeding occurs throughout urination, the disorder is located above the bladder neck. Hematuria can also be caused by GI, vaginal, or certain coagulation disorders.

Urinary frequency, urgency, and hesitancy

An increased urge to urinate commonly results from decreased bladder capacity and is a classic symptom of a UTI. Frequency also occurs with urethral stricture, neurologic disorders, pregnancy, and uterine tumors.

It's a pain

In many cases, the sudden urge to urinate is accompanied by bladder pain and is another symptom of a UTI. Even small amounts of urine in the bladder can cause pain because inflammation decreases bladder capacity. Urgency without pain may be a symptom of an upper motor neuron lesion that affects bladder control.

Difficulty starting a urine stream can occur with a UTI, a partial obstruction of the lower urinary tract, neuromuscular disorders, or the use of certain drugs.

Nocturia

Excessive urination at night, or nocturia, is a common sign of kidney or lower urinary tract disorders. It can result from a disruption of the normal urine patterns or from overstimulation of the nerves and muscles that control urination. It may also be caused by cardiovascular, endocrine, or metabolic disorders and is a common adverse effect of diuretics.

Urinary incontinence

Urinary incontinence is a common complaint that may be transient or permanent. The amount of urine released may be small or large. Possible causes include stress incontinence, tumor, bladder cancer or calculi, and neurologic disorders such as Guillain-Barré syndrome, multiple sclerosis, and spinal cord injury.

Dysuria

Dysuria, or pain during urination, signals a lower UTI. The onset of pain suggests the cause of dysuria. For example, pain just before urination indicates bladder irritation or distension. Pain at the start of urination usually signals a bladder outlet obstruction. Pain at the end of urination can be a sign of bladder spasm, and pain throughout urination may indicate pyelonephrosis, especially when fever, chills, hematuria, and flank pain are also present.

Genital abnormalities

Common female genital abnormalities include genital lesions, vaginal inflammation and discharge, cervical lesions and polyps, vaginal and uterine prolapse, and rectocele.

Genital lesions

In the early stages, syphilitic chancre causes a painless, eroding lesion with a raised, indurated border. The lesion usually appears inside the vagina, but it may also appear on the external genitalia.

Genital warts, a sexually transmitted disease caused by human papillomavirus, produces painless warts on the vulva, vagina, and cervix. Warts start as tiny red or pink swellings that grow and develop stemlike structures. Multiple swellings with a cauliflower appearance are common.

Herpes breakdown

Genital herpes produces multiple, shallow vesicles, lesions, or crusts inside the vagina, on the external genitalia, on the buttocks, and sometimes on the thighs. Dysuria, regional lymph node inflammation, pain, edema, and fever may be present. A Pap test reveals multinucleated giant cells with intranuclear inclusion bodies.

Vaginal inflammation and discharge

Vaginitis usually results from an overgrowth of infectious organisms. It causes redness, itching, dyspareunia (painful intercourse), dysuria, and a malodorous discharge. Bacterial vaginosis causes a fishy odor and a thin, grayish white discharge. *Candida albicans* causes pruritus and a thick, white, curdlike discharge that appears in patches on the cervix and vaginal walls. The discharge has a yeastlike odor.

Effects of STDs

Trichomoniasis may cause an abundant malodorous discharge that's either yellow or green and frothy or watery. It is transmitted sexually. Besides redness, you may note red papules on the cervix and vaginal walls.

A common but in many cases subtle STD, *Chlamydia trachomatis* causes a mucopurulent cervical discharge and cystitis. Gonorrhea is commonly asymptomatic, but it may cause a purulent green-yellow discharge and cystitis.

Cervical lesions and polyps

During a speculum examination, you may detect late-stage cervical cancer as hard, granular, friable lesions; in the early stages, the cervix looks normal. Cervical polyps are bright red, soft, and fragile. They're usually benign, but they may bleed. They usually arise from the endocervical canal.

Cervical cyanosis

Cervical cyanosis may accompany any disorder that causes systemic hypoxia or venous congestion in the cervix. It is also common during pregnancy.

Vaginal and uterine prolapse

Also called cystocele, vaginal prolapse occurs when the anterior vaginal wall and bladder prolapse into the vagina. During speculum examination, you'll see a pouch or bulging on the anterior wall as the patient bears down. The uterus also may prolapse into the vagina and even be visible outside the body.

Rectocele

Rectocele is the herniation of the rectum through the posterior vaginal wall. On examination, you'll see a pouch or bulging on the posterior wall as the patient bears down.

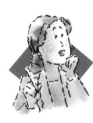

Quick quiz

1. Your patient complains of a thick, white vaginal discharge and vaginal itch. You suspect:
    A. gonorrhea.
    B. *Candida albicans.*
    C. bacterial vaginosis.

Answer: B. *Candida albicans,* or yeast infection, causes pruritus and a thick, white, curdlike discharge with a yeastlike odor that appears in patches on the cervix and vaginal walls.

2. Your patient complains of lower abdominal pressure, and you note a firm mass extending above the symphysis pubis. You suspect:
    A. a distended bladder.
    B. an enlarged kidney.
    C. a UTI.

Answer: A. The bladder is usually nonpalpable unless it's distended. The feeling of pressure is usually relieved with urination.

3. The ducts of Skene's glands open into the:
    A. vulva.
    B. clitoris.
    C. urethra.

Answer: A. Skene's glands are multiple, tiny structures located just below the urethra, each containing 6 to 31 ducts that empty into the vulva.

4. Your patient reports a 32-day menstrual cycle. You know this cycle is probably:
    A. a normal variation.
    B. a sign of metrorrhagia.
    C. a precursor to uterine cancer.

Answer: A. The menstrual cycle varies from woman to woman. If a woman's pattern changes, she should be evaluated further.

5. Using commercial lubricants on speculum blades before inserting them into the vagina should be avoided because:
    A. lubricants can alter test results.
    B. additional lubrication is unnecessary.
    C. many patients are hypersensitive to lubricants.

Answer: A. Most commercial lubricants are bacteriostatic and can alter test and culture results. Hold the speculum blades under warm running water to lubricate them.

6. Your teenage patient complains of a perineal sore. You suspect:
    A. herpes.
    B. chlamydia.
    C. gonorrhea.

Answer: A. Herpes causes multiple shallow vesicles, lesions, or crusts inside the vagina, on the external genitalia, on the buttocks, and sometimes on the thighs.

Scoring

✰✰✰   If you answered all six items correctly, fantastic! You're the new Chancellor of the College of Reproductive Disorders!

✰✰   If you answered four or five correctly, excellent! You're the new Dean of the School of Urinary System Disorders!

✰   If you answered fewer than four correctly, keep at it. Soon, you'll be the new program coordinator for the School of Kidney Percussion!

Male genitourinary system

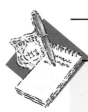

Just the facts

This chapter reviews the male genitourinary (GU) system and how it differs from the female GU system. (For general information about the urinary system, see Chapter 11.) In this chapter, you'll learn:

♦ how to identify the organs and structures of the male GU system

♦ how to obtain a patient history about the male GU system

♦ how to conduct a physical assessment of the male GU system

♦ what causes male GU system abnormalities and how to recognize them.

A look at the male GU system

A disorder of the male urinary or reproductive system can have far-reaching consequences. Besides affecting the system itself, such a disorder can trigger problems in other body systems as well. It also can affect the patient's quality of life, self-esteem, and sense of well-being.

Despite these implications, many men are reluctant to discuss their problems with a nurse or to have intimate areas of their bodies examined. Your challenge, then, is to perform an assessment that's both skilled and sensitive. To do this, you need to be aware of your own feelings about sexuality. If you appear comfortable discussing the patient's problem, he'll be encouraged to talk openly, too.

To thoroughly and accurately assess your patient's GU system, you'll need to review the urinary and reproductive systems' organs and structures and how they work.

Urinary system

The urinary system helps maintain homeostasis by regulating fluid and electrolyte balance. It consists of the kidneys, ureters, bladder, and urethra. The essential functions of the system, such as forming urine and maintaining homeostasis, take place in the highly vascular kidneys.

Much longer urethra

Although the male and female urinary systems function in the same way, a man's urethra is 8″ (20.3 cm) long — about 6″ (15.2 cm) longer than a woman's. That's because it must pass through the erectile tissue of the penis.

Reproductive system

In men, the urethra is also part of the reproductive system, carrying semen as well as urine. (See *Male reproductive system.*) The male reproductive system also includes the penis, scrotum, testicles, epididymis, vas deferens, seminal vesicles, and prostate gland.

Penis

The penis consists of the shaft, glans, urethral meatus, corona, and prepuce. The skin of the penis is hairless and usually darker than the skin on other parts of the body.

The shaft contains three columns of vascular erectile tissue. The glans is located at the end of the penis. The urethral meatus — a slitlike opening — is located ventrally at the tip of the glans. The corona is formed by the junction of the glans and the shaft. The prepuce, the loose skin covering the glans, is often surgically removed shortly after birth in a procedure called circumcision.

When the penile tissues are engorged with blood, the erect penis can discharge sperm. During sexual activity, sperm and semen are forcefully ejaculated from the urethral meatus.

Scrotum

A loose, wrinkled, deeply pigmented pouch, the scrotum is located at the base of the penis. It consists of a muscle layer covered by thin skin and is divided into two compart-

Male reproductive system

This illustration shows the important structures of the male reproductive system

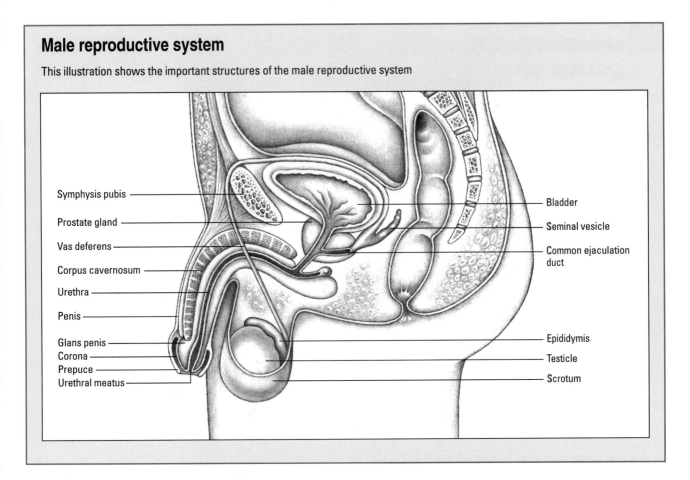

Symphysis pubis

Prostate gland

Vas deferens

Corpus cavernosum

Urethra

Penis

Glans penis

Corona

Prepuce

Urethral meatus

Bladder

Seminal vesicle

Common ejaculation duct

Epididymis

Testicle

Scrotum

ments. Each compartment contains a testicle, epididymis, and portions of the spermatic cord. The left side of the scrotum is usually lower than the right because the left spermatic cord is longer.

Testicles

The testicles are oval, rubbery structures suspended vertically and slightly forward in the scrotum. They produce testosterone and sperm.

Testosterone stimulates the changes that occur during puberty, which starts between ages 9½ and 13½. The testicles enlarge, pubic hair grows, and penis size increases. Secondary sex characteristics appear, such as facial and body hair, muscle development, and voice changes.

Epididymis

The epididymis is a reservoir for maturing sperm. It curves over the posterolateral surface of each testicle, creating a visible bulge on the surface. In a small number of men, the epididymis is located anteriorly.

Vas deferens

The vas deferens — a storage site and the pathway for sperm — begins at the lower end of the epididymis, climbs the spermatic cord, travels through the inguinal canal, and ends in the abdominal cavity where it lies on the fundus of the bladder.

Seminal vesicles

A pair of saclike glands, the seminal vesicles are found on the lower posterior surface of the bladder in front of the rectum. Secretions from the seminal vesicles help form seminal fluid.

Prostate gland

A walnut-shaped gland about 2½" (6.5 cm) long, the prostate surrounds the urethra like a doughnut, just below the bladder. It produces a thin, milky, alkaline fluid that mixes with seminal fluid during ejaculation to enhance sperm activity.

Obtaining a health history

Common complaints about the urinary system include pain during urination and changes in urine output, voiding pattern, and urine color. The most common complaints about the reproductive system are penile discharge, impotence, infertility, and scrotal or inguinal masses, pain, and tenderness.

As you obtain a health history, remember that the patient may feel uncomfortable discussing urinary or reproductive problems. (See *Putting your patient at ease*.)

Ask about past health and family health

Ask the patient about his medical history, especially the presence of diabetes or hypertension. Has he ever had a kidney or bladder infection or an infection of the reproductive system? (See *Assessing urine appearance*.) How about

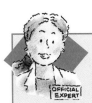

Advice from the experts

Putting your patient at ease

Here are some tips for helping your patient feel more comfortable during the health history.

☑ Make sure the room is private and that you won't be interrupted.

☑ Phrase your questions clearly and tactfully.

☑ Tell the patient that his answers will remain confidential.

☑ Start with less sensitive areas such as urinary function, and work up to more sensitive areas such as sexual function.

☑ Don't rush or omit important facts because the patient seems embarrassed.

☑ Be especially tactful with older men, who may see a normal decrease in sexual prowess as a sign of declining health. They may also be more reluctant to talk about sexual problems than younger men.

☑ When asking questions, keep in mind that many men view sexual problems as a sign of diminished masculinity. So phrase your questions carefully and offer reassurance, as needed.

☑ Consider the patient's educational and cultural background. If he uses slang or euphemisms to talk about his sexual organs or sexual function, make sure you're both talking about the same thing.

kidney or bladder trauma or kidney stones? Has he ever been catheterized?

Also inquire about his family's health to get information on his risk of developing renal failure or kidney disease.

Ask about current health

Ask the patient if he's circumcised. If not, can he retract and replace the prepuce easily? An inability to retract the prepuce is called phimosis; an inability to replace it is called paraphimosis. Untreated, these conditions can impair local circulation and lead to edema and even gangrene.

Inquire whether he has noticed sores, lumps, or ulcers on his penis. These can signal a sexually transmitted disease (STD). Does he have scrotal swelling? This can indicate an inguinal hernia, a hematocele, epididymitis, or a testicular tumor. Also ask if he has penile discharge or bleeding.

Assessing urine appearance

How your patient's urine looks can provide important clues about his general health and the source of his genitourinary problem. During the health history, ask him if he's noticed any changes from the normal straw color. If he has, use this list to help interpret the changes.

• Pale, dilute appearance — diabetes insipidus, diuretic therapy, excessive fluid intake
• Dark yellow or amber, concentrated appearance — acute febrile disease, inadequate fluids, severe diarrhea or vomiting
• Blue-green — methylene blue ingestion
• Green-brown — bile duct obstruction
• Dark brown or black — acute glomerulonephritis, drugs such as chlorpromazine
• Orange-red or orange-brown — obstructive jaundice, urobilinuria, or drugs such as rifampin or phenazopyridine
• Red or red-brown — drugs such as phenazopyridine, hemorrhage, porphyria

Ask about medications

Ask what medications the patient regularly takes. Some drugs can affect the appearance of urine or alter GU function.

Ask about sexual health and practices

Finally, ask the patient about his sexual preference and practices to assess risk-taking behaviors. How many sexual partners does he currently have? Has he ever had an STD? What precautions does he take to prevent contracting STDs? What is his human immunodeficiency virus status?

Also ask about his sexual health. Has he ever been diagnosed with a low sperm count? If so, caution him that hot baths, frequent bicycle riding, and tight underwear or athletic supporters can elevate scrotal temperature and temporarily decrease sperm count. If he participates in sports, ask how he protects himself from possible genital injuries. This is also a good time to ask him if he knows how to examine his testicles for signs of testicular cancer. (See *Testicular self-examination*.)

Assessing the male GU system

To perform a physical assessment of the male GU system, use the techniques of inspection, percussion, palpation, and auscultation. Assessment of the urinary system may be done now or as part of the gastrointestinal assessment.

Examining the urinary system

In many ways, assessing the male urinary system is similar to assessing the female urinary system. Before examining specific structures, check the patient's blood pressure and weight.

Scan the skin

Also observe the patient's skin. A person with decreased renal function may be pale because of a low hemoglobin level or may even have uremic frost — snowlike crystals on the skin from metabolic wastes. In addition, look for signs of fluid imbalance, such as dry mucous membranes, sunken eyeballs, edema, or ascites.

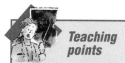

Teaching points

Testicular self-examination

During the patient history, ask your patient if he performs monthly testicular self-examinations. If he doesn't, explain that testicular cancer, the most common cancer in men ages 20 to 35, can be treated successfully when it's detected early.

Teach this technique
To do the examination, the patient should roll each testicle between his thumb and first two fingers. A normal testicle should be free of lumps, move freely in the scrotal sac, and feel firm, smooth, and rubbery. Both testicles should be the same size, although the left one is usually lower than the right because the left spermatic cord is longer.

Before performing an assessment, ask the patient to urinate; then help him into the supine position with his arms at his sides. As you proceed, expose only the areas being examined.

Inspection

First, inspect the patient's abdomen. When he's supine, his abdomen should be smooth, flat or concave, and symmetrical. The skin should be free of lesions, bruises, discolorations, and prominent veins.

Silvery streaks of striae

Watch for abdominal distention with tight, glistening skin and striae — silvery streaks caused by rapidly developing skin tension. These are signs of ascites, which may accompany nephrotic syndrome. This syndrome is characterized by edema, increased urine protein levels, and decreased serum albumin levels.

Percussion and palpation

Percuss the kidneys, checking for pain or tenderness. (See *Performing fist percussion.*) Then percuss the bladder to elicit tympany or dullness. Be sure to tell the patient what you're going to do; otherwise, he may be startled, and you could mistake his reaction for a feeling of acute tenderness. Pain or tenderness suggests a kidney infection.

Hear both sides of the story

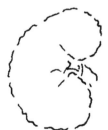

Remember to percuss both sides of the body to assess both kidneys. A dull sound instead of the normal tympany may indicate retained urine in the bladder caused by bladder dysfunction or infection. You can also palpate the kidneys and bladder.

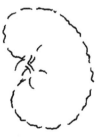

Auscultation

Auscultate the renal arteries to rule out bruits, which signal renal artery stenosis. You can perform this now or as part of an abdominal assessment.

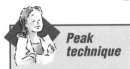

Peak technique

Performing fist percussion

To assess the kidneys by indirect fist percussion, ask the patient to sit up with his back to you. Place one hand at the costovertebral angle and strike it with the ulnar surface of your other hand, as shown.

Costovertebral angle

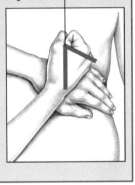

Examining the reproductive system

Before examining the reproductive system, put on gloves. Make the patient as comfortable as possible, and explain what you're doing every step of the way. This will help the patient feel less embarrassed.

Inspection

Inspect the penis, scrotum and testicles, and inguinal and femoral areas.

Penis

Start by examining the penis. Penis size depends on the patient's age and overall development. The penile skin should be slightly wrinkled and pink to light brown in Whites and light brown to dark brown in Blacks. Check the penile shaft and glans for lesions, nodules, inflammation, and swelling. Also check the glans for smegma, a cheesy secretion commonly found beneath the prepuce.

Then gently compress the tip of the glans to open the urethral meatus. (See *Examining the urethral meatus.*) It should be located in the center of the glans and be pink and smooth. Inspect it for swelling, discharge, lesions, inflammation and, especially, genital warts. If you note discharge, obtain a culture specimen.

Scrotum and testicles

Have the patient hold his penis away from his scrotum so you can observe the scrotum's general size and appearance. The skin here is darker than on the rest of the body. Spread the surface of the scrotum, and examine the skin for swelling, nodules, redness, ulceration, and distended veins.

Sebaceous cysts — firm, white to yellow, nontender cutaneous lesions — are a normal finding. Also, check for pitting edema, a sign of cardiovascular disease. Spread the pubic hair and check the skin for lesions and parasites. If the patient is a child, check especially for penile enlargement. (See *Assessing pediatric patients.*)

Inguinal and femoral areas

Have the patient stand. Then ask him to hold his breath and bear down while you inspect the inguinal and femoral

Examining the urethral meatus

To inspect the urethral meatus, compress the tip of the glans, as shown.

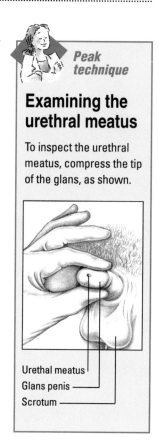

Urethal meatus
Glans penis
Scrotum

areas for bulges or hernias. A hernia is a loop of bowel that comes through a muscle wall.

Palpation

Palpate the penis, testicles, epididymis, spermatic cords, inguinal and femoral areas, and prostate gland.

Penis

Use your thumb and forefinger to palpate the entire penile shaft. It should be somewhat firm, and the skin should be smooth and movable. Note swelling, nodules, or indurations.

Testicles

Gently palpate both testicles between your thumb and first two fingers. Assess their size, shape, and response to pressure. A normal response is a deep visceral pain. The testicles should be equal in size, move freely in the scrotal sac, and feel firm, smooth, and rubbery.

If you note hard, irregular areas or lumps, transilluminate them by darkening the room and pressing the head of a flashlight against the scrotum, behind the lump. The testicle and any lumps, masses, warts, or blood-filled areas will appear as opaque shadows.

Transilluminate the other testicle to compare your findings. This is also a good time to reinforce the methods and importance of doing a monthly testicular self-examination.

Epididymis

Next, palpate the epididymis, which is usually located in the posterolateral area of the testicle. It should be smooth, discrete, nontender, and free of swelling or induration.

Spermatic cords

Palpate both spermatic cords, which are located above each testicle. Palpate from the base of the epididymis to the inguinal canal. The vas deferens is a smooth, movable cord inside the spermatic cord. If you feel swelling, irregularity, or nodules, transilluminate the problem area, as described above. If serous fluid is present, you'll see a red glow; if tissue and blood are present, you won't see this glow.

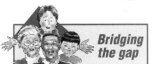

Bridging the gap

Assessing pediatric patients

Before palpating a boy's scrotum for a testicular examination, explain what you'll be doing and why. Make sure he's comfortably warm and as relaxed as possible. Cold and anxiety may cause his testicles to retract so that you can't palpate them.

Hernias and hydroceles

If you see an enlarged scrotum in a boy younger than age 2, suspect a scrotal extension of an inguinal hernia, a hydrocele, or both. Hydroceles, often associated with inguinal hernias, are common in children of this age-group. To differentiate between the two, remember that hydroceles transilluminate and aren't tender or reducible.

Obesity

An adolescent boy who's obese may appear to have an abnormally small penis. You may have to retract the fat over the symphysis pubis to properly assess penis size.

Inguinal area

To assess for a direct inguinal hernia, place two fingers over each external inguinal ring, and ask the patient to bear down. If he has a hernia, you'll feel a bulge.

To assess for an indirect inguinal hernia, examine the patient while he's standing and then while he's supine with his knee flexed on the side you're examining. (See *Palpating for an indirect inguinal hernia*.)

Place your index finger on the neck of the scrotum and gently push upward into the inguinal canal. When you've inserted your finger as far as possible, ask the patient to bear down or cough. A hernia feels like a mass of tissue that withdraws when met by the finger.

Femoral area

Although you can't palpate the femoral canal, you can estimate its location to help detect a femoral hernia. Place your right index finger on the right femoral artery with your finger pointing toward the patient's head. Keep your other fingers close together. Your middle finger will lie over the femoral vein, and your ring finger will lie over the femoral canal. Note tenderness or masses. Use your left hand to check the patient's left side.

Prostate gland

Warn the patient that he'll feel some pressure or urgency during this examination. Have him stand and lean over the examination table. If he can't do this, have him lie on his left side, with his right knee and hip flexed or with both knees drawn toward his chest. Inspect the skin of the perineal, anal, and posterior scrotal areas. It should be smooth and unbroken with no protruding masses.

Then lubricate the gloved index finger of your dominant hand and insert it into the rectum. Tell the patient to relax to ease passage of the finger through the anal sphincter. With your finger pad, palpate the prostate gland on the anterior rectal wall just past the anorectal ring. (See *Palpating the prostate gland*.) The gland should feel smooth, rubbery, and about the size of a walnut.

If it protrudes into the rectal lumen, it's probably enlarged. An enlarged prostate gland is classified as grade 1 (protruding less than ⅜″ [1 cm] into the rectal lumen) to grade 4 (protruding more than 1¼″ [3.2 cm] into the rectal lumen). Also note tenderness or nodules.

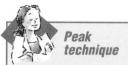

Peak technique

Palpating for an indirect inguinal hernia

To palpate for an indirect inguinal hernia, place your gloved finger on the neck of the scrotum and insert it into the inguinal canal, as shown. Then ask the patient to bear down.

If the patient has a hernia, you'll feel a soft mass at your fingertip.

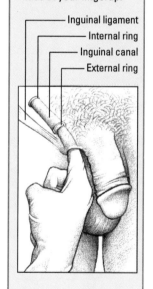

— Inguinal ligament
— Internal ring
— Inguinal canal
— External ring

Abnormal findings

Your assessment may uncover abnormalities of the GU system. Although the urinary problems below also occur in women, the causes described are unique to the male patient.

Urinary problems

Hematuria

A patient with hematuria may have brown or bright-red urine. Bleeding at the end of urination signals a disorder of the bladder neck, posterior urethra, or prostate gland.

Urinary frequency, urgency, and hesitancy

Urinary frequency and urgency are classic symptoms of a urinary tract infection (UTI). Urinary frequency also occurs with benign prostatic hyperplasia, urethral stricture, and a prostate tumor, which can put pressure on the bladder.

Urinary hesitancy is most common in older men who have prostatic enlargement, which causes partial obstruction of the urethra.

Nocturia

Excessive urination at night, or nocturia, is a common sign of renal or lower urinary tract disorders. It can result from benign prostatic hypertrophy, when significant urethral obstruction develops, or from prostate cancer.

Urinary incontinence

Urinary incontinence may be caused by benign prostatic hypertrophy, prostate infection, and prostate cancer.

Reproductive system problems

Penile lesions

Lesions on the penis can vary in appearance. (See *Male genital lesions,* page 250.) A hard, nontender nodule, especially on the glans or inner lip of the prepuce, may indicate carcinoma of the penis.

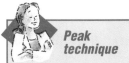

Peak technique

Palpating the prostate gland

To palpate the prostate gland, insert your gloved, lubricated index finger into the rectum. Then palpate the prostate on the anterior rectal wall, just past the anorectal ring, as shown.

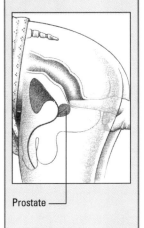

Prostate

Male genital lesions

Several types of lesions may affect the male genitalia. Some of the more common ones are described below.

Penile cancer causes a painless, ulcerative lesion on the glans or foreskin, possibly accompanied by discharge.

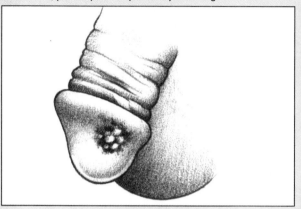

Genital herpes causes a painful, reddened group of small vesicles or blisters on the foreskin, shaft, or glans. Lesions eventually disappear but tend to recur.

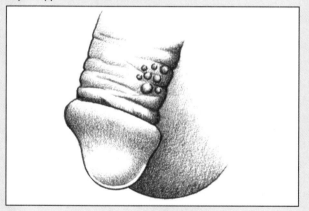

Genital warts are flesh-colored papillary growths that occur singly or in cauliflowerlike clusters. They may be barely visible or several inches in diameter.

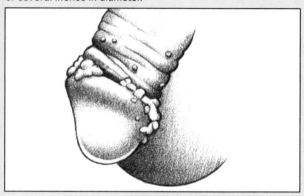

Syphilis causes a hard, round papule — usually on the glans penis. When palpated, this syphilitic chancre may feel like a button. Eventually, the papule erodes into an ulcer. You may also note swollen lymph nodes in the inguinal area.

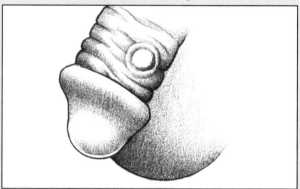

Penile discharge

A profuse, yellow discharge from the penis suggests gonococcal urethritis. Other symptoms may include urinary frequency, burning, and urgency. Without treatment, the prostate gland, epididymis, and periurethral glands will become inflamed. A copious, watery, purulent urethral discharge may indicate chlamydial infection. Bloody discharge can mean infection or cancer in the urinary or reproductive tract.

Paraphimosis

In paraphimosis, the prepuce is so tight that, when retracted, it gets caught behind the glans and can't be replaced. Edema can result. Instruct uncircumcised men to retract the prepuce each time they clean the glans, and then to replace it afterward. Frequent retraction and cleaning prevents excessive tightness of the prepuce, which in turn prevents the prepuce from closing off the urinary meatus and constricting the glans.

Displacement of the urethral meatus

When the urethral meatus is located on the underside of the penis, the condition is called hypospadias. When it's on the top of the urethral meatus, it's called epispadias. Both conditions are congenital.

Testicular tumor

A painless scrotal nodule that can't be transilluminated may be a testicular tumor. This disorder occurs most often in men ages 20 to 35. The tumor can grow, enlarging the testicle.

Hydrocele

An enlarged scrotum may be a sign of a hydrocele, or a collection of fluid in the testicle. Hydrocele is associated with conditions that cause poor fluid reabsorption, such as cirrhosis, congestive heart failure, and testicular tumor. A hydrocele can be transilluminated.

Hernias

A direct inguinal hernia emerges from behind the external inguinal ring and protrudes through it. It seldom descends into the scrotum and usually affects men over age 40.

An indirect inguinal hernia can be palpated in the internal inguinal canal with its tip in or beyond the canal. Or it may descend into the scrotum. An indirect inguinal hernia, the most common type of hernia, occurs in men of all ages.

A femoral hernia feels like a soft tumor below the inguinal ligament in the femoral area. It may be difficult to distinguish from a lymph node and is uncommon in men.

Prostate gland enlargement

A smooth, firm, symmetrical enlargement of the prostate gland indicates benign prostatic hypertrophy, which typically starts in the fifth decade of life. This finding may be associated with nocturia, urinary hesitancy and frequency, and recurring UTIs.

Prostate cancer

Hard, irregular, fixed lesions that make the prostate feel asymmetrical suggest prostate cancer. Palpation may or may not be painful. This condition also causes urinary dysfunction. Back and leg pain may occur with bone metastases in advanced stages.

Acute prostatitis

In acute prostatitis, the prostate gland is firm, warm, and extremely tender and swollen. Because this condition is caused by a bacterial infection, the patient usually has a fever.

Memory jogger

To help you remember what findings suggest prostate cancer, think of the word PAINS.

P   prostate cancer

A   asymmetric

I   irregular

N   nodules

S   stony (hard) and fixed

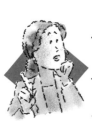

Quick quiz

1. Stress to the patient the importance of self-examination of the testicles every:
   A. day.
   B. week.
   C. month.

Answer: C. A monthly testicular self-examination can help detect testicular cancer early.

2. An inguinal hernia is best palpated with the patient:
   A. sitting.
   B. supine.
   C. standing.

Answer: C. To check for an inguinal hernia, have the patient stand and then hold his breath and bear down while you palpate the area.

3. Signs of benign prostatic hypertrophy include:
   A. an irregular, pea-shaped gland.
   B. an enlarged, hard gland with asymmetric swelling.
   C. a smooth, firm, symmetrical enlargement of the prostate gland.

Answer: C. In men over age 50, a smooth, firm, symmetrical enlargement of the prostate gland may be a normal finding.

4. Although the male and female urinary systems function in the same way, there is a difference in the length of the:
   A. urethra.
   B. ureter.
   C. epididymis.

Answer: A. Because a man's urethra passes through the erectile tissue of the penis, it's about 6″ (15 cm) longer than a woman's. A man's urethra carries semen as well as urine.

5. You would expect the skin of a patient with decreased renal function to be:
   A. dry and cracked.
   B. bruised and discolored.
   C. pale and covered with uremic frost.

Answer: C. Decreased renal function may cause pale skin, due to a low hemoglobin level, and uremic frost — snow-like crystals from metabolic wastes.

6. Treatment for paraphimosis includes:
   A. applying warmth to the testicles.
   B. replacing the prepuce over the glans.
   C corticosteroid injections of the vas deferens.

Answer: B. In paraphimosis, the prepuce is so tight that when it's retracted, it gets caught behind the glans and can't be replaced. Treatment consists in part of replacing the prepuce over the glans.

Scoring

☆☆☆ If you answered all six items correctly, look up to the sky! You're the galaxy's brightest nursing star!

☆☆ If you answered four or five items correctly, congratulations! You're more dazzling than a meteor shower!

☆ If you answered fewer than four items correctly, that's great! You're exploring a new universe of assessment skills.

Musculoskeletal system

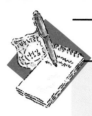

Just the facts

This chapter describes the musculoskeletal system, which includes joints, bones, and muscles. In this chapter, you'll learn:

♦ how to identify structures of the musculoskeletal system

♦ questions to ask during a health history

♦ how to use inspection and palpation to assess the musculoskeletal system

♦ how to identify disorders of the musculoskeletal system

♦ how to identify abnormal findings and understand their significance.

A look at the musculoskeletal system

During a musculoskeletal assessment, you'll use your senses of sight, hearing, and touch to determine the health of the patient's muscles, bones, joints, tendons, and ligaments. These structures give the human body its shape and ability to move. Your sharp assessment skills will help uncover musculoskeletal abnormalities and evaluate the patient's ability to perform activities of daily living.

The three main parts of the musculoskeletal system are the bones, joints, and muscles.

Bones

The 206 bones of the skeleton form the body's framework, supporting organs and tissues. (See *A close look at the skeletal system*.) The bones also serve as storage sites for minerals and produce blood cells.

A close look at the skeletal system

Of the 206 bones in the human skeletal system, 80 form the axial skeleton, or head and trunk, and 126 form the appendicular skeleton, or the extremities. Shown below are the body's major bones.

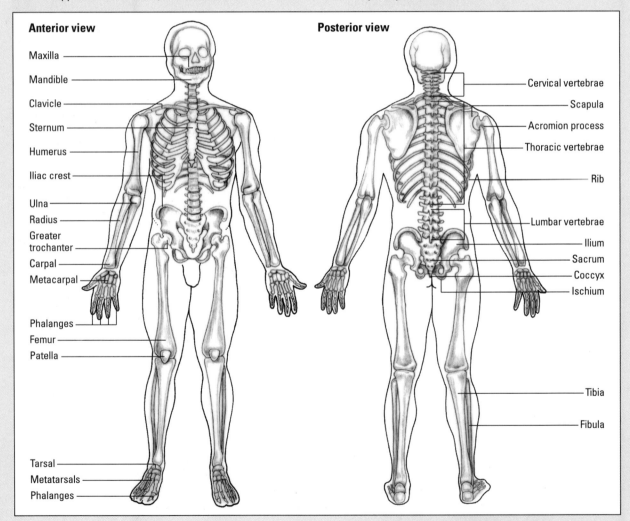

Anterior view

- Maxilla
- Mandible
- Clavicle
- Sternum
- Humerus
- Iliac crest
- Ulna
- Radius
- Greater trochanter
- Carpal
- Metacarpal
- Phalanges
- Femur
- Patella
- Tarsal
- Metatarsals
- Phalanges

Posterior view

- Cervical vertebrae
- Scapula
- Acromion process
- Thoracic vertebrae
- Rib
- Lumbar vertebrae
- Ilium
- Sacrum
- Coccyx
- Ischium
- Tibia
- Fibula

Joints

The junction of two or more bones is called a joint. Joints stabilize the bones and allow a specific type of movement. The two types of joints are nonsynovial and synovial. In nonsynovial joints, the bones are connected by fibrous tissue or cartilage. The bones may be immovable, like the sutures in the skull, or slightly movable, like the vertebrae.

Synovial joints move freely; the bones are separate from each other and meet in a cavity filled with synovial fluid, a lubricant. (See *Synovial joint*.)

In synovial joints, a layer of resilient cartilage covers the surfaces of opposing bones. This cartilage cushions the bones and allows full joint movement by making the surfaces of the bones smooth. (See *Types of joint motion*, page 258.)

Some popular joints

Synovial joints come in several types, including ball-and-socket joints and hinge joints.

The only ball-and-socket joints in the body — the shoulder and hip — allow for flexion, extension, adduction, and abduction. These joints also rotate in their sockets and are assessed by their degree of internal and external rotation.

Hinge joints, such as the knee and elbow, normally move in flexion and extension only.

They're surrounded

Synovial joints are surrounded by a fibrous capsule that stabilizes the joint structures. The capsule also surrounds the joint's ligaments — the tough, fibrous bands that join one bone to another.

Muscles

Skeletal muscles are groups of contractile cells or fibers. These fibers contract after a stimulus from the central nervous system (CNS), producing skeletal movement. The CNS is responsible for both involuntary and voluntary muscle function.

Tendons are tough fibrous portions of muscle that attach the muscles to bone. Bursae, sacs filled with friction-

Synovial joint

Normally, bones fit together. Cartilage — a smooth, fibrous tissue — cushions the end of each bone, and synovial fluid fills the joint space. This fluid lubricates the joint and eases movement, much as the brake fluid functions in a car.

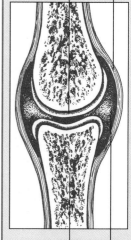

Joint capsule

Cartilage

Bone

Joint space filled with synovial fluid

Types of joint motion

The illustrations below show various areas of the body and what types of movements their joints allow.

Circumduction
Moving in a circular manner

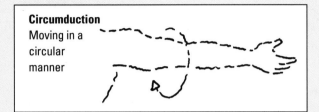

Retraction and protraction
Moving backward and forward

Pronation
Turning downward

Supination
Turning upward

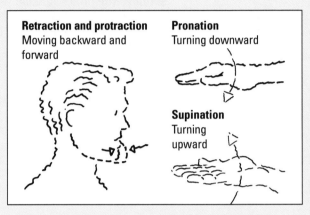

Flexion
Bending, decreasing the joint angle

Extension
Straightening, increasing the joint angle

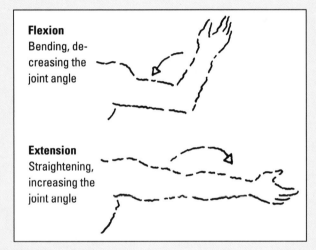

Internal rotation
Turning toward midline

External rotation
Turning away from midline

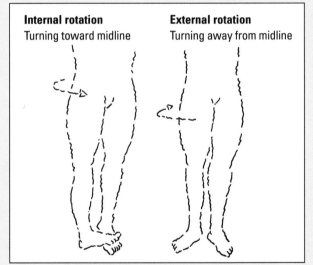

Abduction
Moving away from midline

Adduction
Moving toward midline

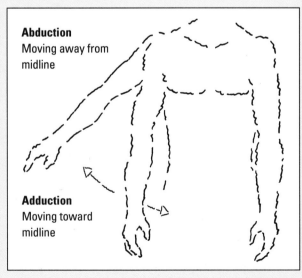

Eversion
Turning outward

Inversion
Turning inward

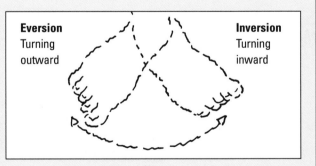

reducing synovial fluid, are located in areas of high friction such as the knee.

Obtaining a health history

The patient's chief complaints are important because they determine the focus of your examination. Patients with joint injuries usually complain of pain, swelling, or stiffness, and they may have noticeable deformities.

Deformity also can occur with a bone fracture, which causes sharp pain when the patient moves the affected area. With a muscular injury, pain, swelling, and weakness are common complaints.

Because many musculoskeletal injuries are emergencies, you might not have time for a thorough assessment. In these cases, the PQRST device explained in Chapter 1 will remind you what key areas to focus on.

Ask about current health

Are the patient's activities of daily living affected? Ask if he has noticed grating sounds when he moves certain parts of his body. Does he use ice, heat, or other remedies to treat the problem?

Ask about past health

Inquire whether the patient has ever had gout, arthritis, tuberculosis, or cancer, which may have bony metastases. Has the patient been diagnosed with osteoporosis?

Ask if he has had a recent blunt or penetrating trauma. If so, how did it happen? For example, did he suffer knee and hip injury after being hit by a car, or did he fall from a ladder and land on his coccyx? This information will help guide your assessment and predict hidden trauma.

Also ask the patient if he uses an assistive device such as a cane, walker, or brace. If so, watch him use the device to assess how he moves.

Ask about medications

Question the patient about what medications he regularly takes. Many drugs can affect the musculoskeletal system. Corticosteroids, for example, can cause muscle weakness, myopathy, osteoporosis, pathologic fractures, and avascular necrosis of the heads of the femur and humerus.

Ask about lifestyle

Ask the patient about his job, hobbies, and personal habits. Knitting, playing football or tennis, working at a computer, or doing construction work can all cause repetitive stress injuries or injure the musculoskeletal system in other ways. Even carrying a heavy knapsack or purse can cause injury or increase muscle size.

Assessing the musculoskeletal system

Because the CNS and the musculoskeletal system are interrelated, you usually should assess them together.

To assess the musculoskeletal system, use the techniques of inspection and palpation to test all the major bones, joints, and muscles. Perform a complete examination if the patient has generalized symptoms such as aching in several joints. Perform an abbreviated examination if he has pain in only one body area such as his ankle.

Go head to toe

Before starting your assessment, have the patient undress down to his underwear and put on a hospital gown. Explain each procedure as you perform it. The only special equipment you'll need is a tape measure.

Begin your examination with a general observation of the patient. Then systematically assess the whole body, working from head to toe and from proximal to distal structures. Because muscles and joints are interdependent, interpret these findings together. As you work your way down the body, follow these general rules:
• Note the size and shape of joints, limbs, and body regions.
• Inspect and palpate the skin and tissues around the joint, limb, or body region for temperature, color, swelling, tenderness, masses, and deformities.
• Have the patient perform active range-of-motion exercises of a joint, if possible. If he can't, use passive range of motion.
• During passive range-of-motion exercises, support the joint firmly on either side and move it gently to avoid causing pain or spasm.

Walk the walk

Whenever possible, observe how the patient stands and moves. Watch him walk into the room or, if he's already in, ask him to walk to the door, turn around, and walk back toward you. His torso should sway only slightly, his arms should swing naturally at his sides, his gait should be even, and his posture should be erect.

As he walks, his foot should flatten and bear his weight completely, and his toes should flex as he pushes off with his foot. In midswing, his foot should clear the floor and pass the other leg.

Assessing the bones and joints

Perform a head-to-toe evaluation of your patient's bones and joints using inspection and palpation. Then perform range-of-motion exercises to help you determine if the joints are healthy.

Head, jaw, and neck

First, inspect the patient's face for swelling, symmetry, and evidence of trauma. The mandible should be in the midline, not shifted to the right or left.

Is the TMJ A-OK?

Next, evaluate range of motion in the temporomandibular joint (TMJ). Place the tips of your first two or three fingers in front of the middle of the ear. Ask the patient to open and close his mouth. Then place your fingers into the depressed area over the joint, and note the motion of the mandible. The patient should be able to open and close his jaw and protract and retract his mandible easily, without pain or tenderness.

If you hear or palpate a click as the patient's mouth opens, suspect an improperly aligned jaw. TMJ dysfunction may also lead to swelling of the area, crepitus, or pain.

Check the neck

Inspect the front, back, and sides of the patient's neck, noting muscle asymmetry or masses. Palpate the spinous processes of the cervical vertebrae and supraclavicular fossae for tenderness, swelling, or nodules.

To palpate the neck area, stand facing the patient with your hands placed lightly on the sides of his neck. Ask him to turn his head from side to side, flex his neck forward, and then extend it backward. Feel for any lumps or tender areas.

As the patient moves his neck, listen and palpate for crepitus. This is an abnormal grating sound, not the occasional "crack" we hear from our joints. (See *What is crepitus?*)

Head circles and chin-ups

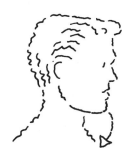

Now, check range of motion in the neck. Ask the patient to try touching his right ear to his right shoulder and his left ear to his left shoulder. The usual range of motion is 40 degrees on each side. Next, ask him to touch his chin to his chest and then to point his chin toward the ceiling. The neck should flex forward 45 degrees and extend backward 55 degrees.

To assess rotation, ask the patient to turn his head to each side without moving his trunk. His chin should be parallel to his shoulders. Finally, ask him to move his head in a circle — normal rotation is 70 degrees.

Spine

Ask the patient to remove the hospital gown so you can observe his spine. First check his spinal curvature as he stands in profile. In this position, the spine has a reverse "S" shape. (See *Kyphosis and lordosis.*)

Next, observe the spine posteriorly. It should be in midline position without deviation to either side. Lateral deviation suggests scoliosis. (See *Testing for scoliosis.*) You also may notice that one shoulder is lower than the other.

To assess for scoliosis, have the patient bend at the waist. This position makes deformities more apparent. Normally, the spine remains at midline.

Does the back measure up?

Next, assess the range of spinal movement. Ask the patient to straighten up, and use the measuring tape to measure the distance from the nape of his neck to his waist. Then ask him to bend forward at the waist. Continue to hold the tape at his neck, letting it slip through your fingers slightly to accommodate the increased distance as the spine flexes.

The length of the spine from neck to waist usually increases by at least 2″(5 cm) when the patient bends for-

---

What is crepitus?

Sometimes a joint makes a cracking sound when it moves. This is a normal sound that occurs when a tendon or ligament slips over bone.

Crepitus is an abnormal finding. It's a crunching or grating you can hear and feel when a joint with roughened articular surfaces moves. It occurs in patients with rheumatoid arthritis or osteoarthritis or when broken pieces of bone rub together.

Kyphosis and lordosis

These illustrations show the difference between kyphosis and lordosis.

Kyphosis
If the patient has a pronounced kyphosis, the thoracic curve is abnormally rounded, as shown.

Lordosis
If the patient has a pronounced lordosis, the lumbar spine is abnormally concave, as shown. Lordosis (as well as a waddling gait) is normal in pregnant women and young children.

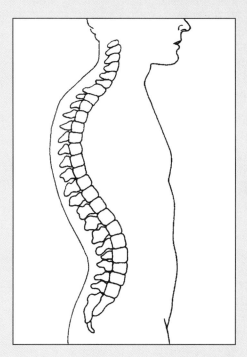

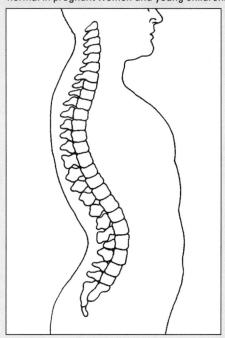

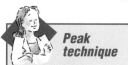

Peak technique

Testing for scoliosis

When testing for scoliosis, have the patient remove her shirt and stand as straight as possible with her back to you. Look for:
• uneven shoulder height and shoulder blade prominence
• unequal distance between the arms and the body
• asymmetrical waistline
• uneven hip height
• sideways lean.

Bent over
Then have her bend forward, keeping her head down and palms together. Look for:
• asymmetrical thoracic spine or prominent rib cage (rib hump) on either side
• asymmetrical waistline.

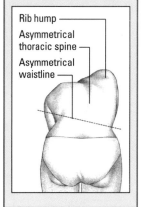

Rib hump

Asymmetrical thoracic spine

Asymmetrical waistline

ward. If it doesn't, the patient's mobility may be impaired, and you'll need to assess him further.

Spine-tingling procedure

Finally, palpate the spinal processes and the areas lateral to the spine. Have the patient bend at the waist and let his arms hang loosely at his sides. Palpate the spine with your fingertips. Then repeat the palpation using the side of your hand, lightly striking the areas lateral to the spine. Note tenderness, swelling, or spasm.

Shoulders and elbows

Start by observing the patient's shoulders, noting asymmetry, muscle atrophy, or deformities. Swelling or loss of the normal rounded shape could mean that one or more bones are dislocated or out of alignment.

Remember, if the patient's chief complaint is shoulder pain, the problem may not have originated in the shoulder. Shoulder pain may be referred from other sources and may be due to a heart attack or ruptured ectopic pregnancy.

Palpate the shoulders with the palmar surfaces of your fingers to locate bony landmarks; note crepitus or tenderness. Using your entire hand, palpate the shoulder muscles for firmness and symmetry of size. Also palpate the elbow and the ulna for subcutaneous nodules that occur with rheumatoid arthritis.

Lift and rotate

If the patient's shoulders don't appear dislocated, assess rotation. Start with the patient's arm straight at his side — the neutral position. Ask him to lift his arm straight up from his side to shoulder level and then to bend his elbow horizontally until his forearm is at a 90-degree angle to his upper arm. His arm should be parallel to the floor, and his fingers should be extended with palms down.

To assess external rotation, have him bring his forearm up until his fingers point toward the ceiling. To assess internal rotation, have him lower his forearm until his fingers point toward the floor. The normal range of motion is 90 degrees in each direction.

Flex and extend

To assess flexion and extension, start with the patient's arm in the neutral position (at his side). To assess flexion, ask him to move his arm anteriorly over his head, as if reaching for the sky. Full flexion is 180 degrees. To assess extension, have him move his arm from the neutral position posteriorly as far as possible. The normal extension range is 30 to 50 degrees.

Swing into position

To assess abduction, ask the patient to move his arm from the neutral position laterally as far as possible. The normal range of motion is 180 degrees.

To assess adduction, have the patient move his arm from the neutral position across the front of his body as far as possible. The normal range of motion is 50 degrees.

He's up to his elbows

Next assess the elbows for flexion and extension. Have the patient rest his arm at his side. Ask him to flex his elbow from this position and then extend it. The normal range of motion is 90 degrees for both flexion and extension.

To assess supination and pronation of the elbow, have the patient place the side of his hand on a flat surface with the thumb on top. Ask him to rotate his palm down toward the table for pronation and upward for supination. The normal angle of elbow rotation is 90 degrees in each direction.

Wrists and hands

Inspect the wrists and hands for contour and compare them for symmetry. Also check for nodules, redness, swelling, deformities, and webbing between the fingers.

Use your thumb and index finger to palpate both wrists and each of the finger joints. Note any tenderness, nodules, or bogginess. To avoid causing pain, be especially gentle with elderly patients and those with arthritis.

Rotate and flap

Assess range of motion in the wrist. Ask the patient to rotate his wrist by moving his entire hand — first laterally and then medially — as if he's waxing a car. The normal range of motion is 55 degrees laterally and 20 degrees medially.

Observe the wrist while the patient extends his fingers up toward the ceiling and down toward the floor, as if he's flapping his hand. He should be able to extend his wrist 70 degrees and flex it 90 degrees. If these movements cause pain or numbness, he may have carpal tunnel syndrome. (See *Testing for carpal tunnel syndrome*, page 266.)

Lift a finger; make a fist

To assess extension and flexion of the metacarpophalangeal joints, ask the patient to keep his wrist still and move only his fingers — first up toward the ceiling and

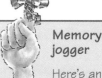

Memory jogger

Here's an easy way to keep adduction and abduction straight. Adduction is moving a limb toward the body's midline; think of it as adding two things together. Abduction is moving a limb away from the body's midline; think of it as taking something away, like abducting or kidnapping.

Peak technique

Testing for carpal tunnel syndrome

Two simple tests — Tinel's signs and Phalen's sign — can confirm carpal tunnel syndrome.

Tinel's sign

Lightly percuss the transverse carpal ligament over the median nerve where the patient's palm and wrist meet. If this action produces discomfort, such as numbness and tingling shooting into the palm and finger, the patient has Tinel's sign and probably has carpal tunnel syndrome.

Phalen's sign

If flexing the patient's wrist for about 30 seconds causes pain or numbness in his hand or fingers, he has Phalen's sign. The more severe the carpal tunnel syndrome, the more rapidly the symptoms develop.

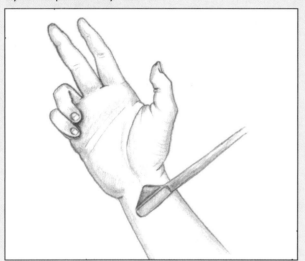

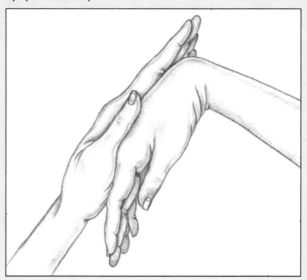

then down toward the floor. Normal findings are 30 degrees of extension and 90 degrees of flexion.

Next, ask the patient to touch his thumb to the little finger of the same hand. He should be able to fold or flex his thumb across the palm of his hand so that it touches or points toward the base of his little finger.

To assess flexion of all of the fingers, ask the patient to form a fist. Then have him spread his fingers apart to demonstrate abduction and draw them back together to demonstrate adduction.

At arm's length

If you suspect that one arm is longer than the other, take measurements. Put one end of the measuring tape at the acromial process of the shoulder and the other on the tip of the middle finger. Drape the tape over the outer elbow. A difference of no more than ⅜″ (1 cm) should exist between the left and right extremities.

Hips and knees

Inspect the hip area for contour and symmetry. Inspect the position of the knees, noting whether the patient is bowlegged, with knees that point out, or knock-kneed, with knees that turn in. Then watch the patient walk.

Palpate both knees. They should feel smooth, and the tissues should feel solid. (See *Bulge sign*.)

Hip, hip, hooray!

Assess hip range of motion. Ideally, these exercises should be done with the patient standing. But if he's elderly or has trouble standing, he can lie supine instead.

To assess hip flexion, have the patient stand and extend his leg forward. He should be able to move his leg forward between 45 and 90 degrees. To assess hip extension, have him return his leg to a straight position (0 de-

Peak technique

Bulge sign

The bulge sign indicates excess fluid in the joint. To assess for this sign, ask the patient to lie down so that you can palpate his knee. Then give the medial side of his knee two to four firm strokes, as shown, to displace excess fluid.

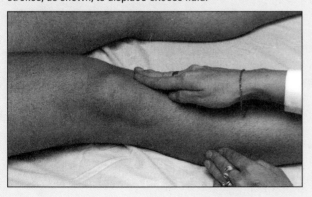

Lateral check

Next, tap the lateral aspect of the knee while checking for a fluid wave on the medial aspect, as shown.

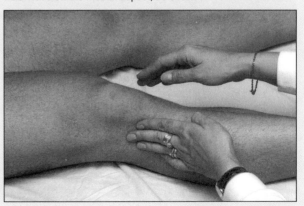

grees). To assess hyperextension, ask him to extend his leg backward keeping his knees straight. He should be able to extend his leg about 30 degrees backward.

Next have him kick out laterally to assess abduction and swing one leg across the other to assess adduction. Normal range of motion is about 45 degrees for abduction and 30 degrees for adduction.

As the hip turns

To assess internal and external rotation of the hip, ask the patient to lift one leg up and, keeping his knee straight, turn his leg and foot medially and laterally. The normal range of motion for internal rotation is 40 degrees and 45 degrees for external rotation.

On bended knees

Assess knee range of motion. If the patient is standing, ask him to bend his knee as if trying to touch his heel to his buttocks. The normal range of motion for flexion is 120 to 130 degrees. If the patient is lying down, have him draw his knee up to his chest. His calf should touch his thigh.

Knee extension returns the knee to a neutral position of 0 degrees. However, some knees may normally be hyperextended 15 degrees. If the patient can't extend his leg fully or if his knee "pops" audibly and painfully, it's abnormal.

Other abnormalities include pronounced crepitus, which may signal a degenerative disease of the knee, and sudden buckling, which may mean a ligament injury.

Ankles and feet

Inspect the ankles and feet for swelling, redness, nodules, and other deformities. Check the arch of the foot and look for toe deformities. Also note edema, calluses, bunions, corns, ingrown toenails, plantar warts, trophic ulcers, hair loss, or unusual pigmentation.

Use your fingertips to palpate the bony and muscular structures of the ankles and feet. Palpate each toe joint by compressing it with your thumb and fingers.

The ankle angle

To examine the ankle, have the patient sit in a chair or on the side of a bed. To test plantar flexion, ask him to point his toes toward the floor. Test dorsiflexion by asking him to point his toes toward the ceiling. The normal range of motion is about 45 degrees for plantar flexion and 20 degrees for dorsiflexion.

Next, assess ankle range of motion. Ask the patient to demonstrate inversion by turning his feet inward and eversion by turning his feet outward. Normal range of motion is 45 degrees for inversion and 30 degrees for eversion.

To assess the metatarsophalangeal joints, ask the patient to flex his toes and then straighten them.

The long and short of it

If you suspect that one leg is longer than the other, take measurements. Put one end of the tape at the medial malleolus at the ankle and the other end at the anterior iliac spine. Cross the tape over the medial side of the knee. A difference of more than ⅜″ (1 cm) is abnormal.

Assessing the muscles

Start by inspecting all major muscle groups for tone, strength, asymmetry, and other abnormalities. If a muscle appears atrophied or hypertrophied, measure it by wrapping a tape measure around the largest circumference of the muscle on each side of the body and then comparing the two numbers.

Other abnormalities of muscle appearance include contracture and abnormal movements, such as spasms, tics, tremors, or fasciculation.

Tuning into muscle tone

Muscle tone describes muscular resistance to passive stretching. To test the patient's arm muscle tone, move his shoulder through passive range-of-motion exercises. You should feel a slight resistance. Then let his arm drop. It should fall easily to his side.

Test leg muscle tone by putting the patient's hip through passive range-of-motion exercises and then letting the leg fall to the examination table or bed. Once again, it should fall easily.

Abnormal findings include muscle rigidity and flaccidity. Rigidity indicates increased muscle tone, possibly caused by an upper motor neuron lesion such as from a stroke. Flaccidity may result from a lower motor neuron lesion.

Peak technique

Testing muscle strength

To test the strength of your patient's arm and ankle muscles, use the techniques shown here.

Biceps strength

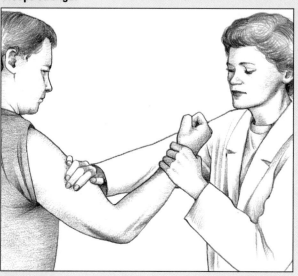

Ankle strength: Plantar flexion

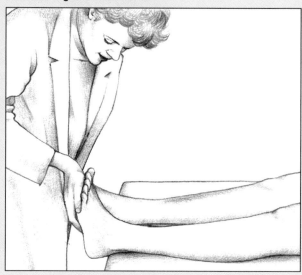

Triceps strength

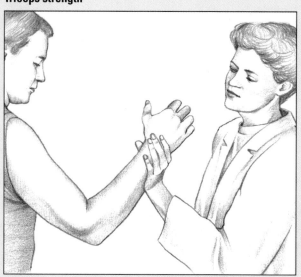

Ankle strength: Dorsiflexion

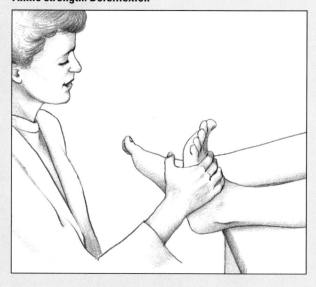

Wrestling with muscle strength

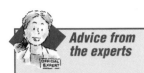
Testing handgrip strength

When testing handgrip strength, face the patient, extend the first and second fingers of each hand, and ask him to grasp your fingers and squeeze. Don't extend fingers with rings on them; a strong handgrip on those fingers can be painful.

Observe the patient's gait and movements to form an idea of his general muscle strength. To test specific muscle groups, ask him to move the muscles while you apply resistance; then compare the contralateral muscle groups. (See *Testing muscle strength*.)

Grade muscle strength on a scale of 0 to 5, with 0 representing no strength and 5 representing maximum strength. (See *Grading muscle strength*.) Document the results as a fraction, with the score as the numerator and maximum strength as the denominator.

Shoulder, arm, wrist, and hand strength

Test the strength of the patient's shoulder girdle by asking him to extend his arms with the palms up and hold this position for 30 seconds. If he can't lift both arms equally and keep his palms up, or if one arm drifts down, he probably has shoulder girdle weakness on that side.

If he passes the first part of the test, gauge his strength by placing your hands on his arms and applying downward pressure as he resists you.

Testing the bi's and tri's

Next, have the patient hold his arm in front of him with the elbow bent. To test biceps strength, pull down on the flexor surface of his forearm as he resists. To test triceps strength, have him try to straighten his arm as you push upward against the extensor surface of his forearm.

Forcing his hand

Assess the strength of the patient's flexed wrist by pushing against it. Test the strength of the extended wrist by pushing down on it. Test the strength of finger abduction, thumb opposition, and handgrip the same way. (See *Testing handgrip strength*.)

Leg strength

Ask the patient to lie supine on the examining table or bed and lift both legs at the same time. Note whether he lifts both legs the same distance. To test quadriceps strength, have him lower his legs and raise them again while you press down on his anterior thighs.

Then ask the patient to flex his knees and put his feet flat on the bed. Assess lower leg strength by pulling his lower leg forward as he resists and then pushing it backward as he extends his knee.

Finally, assess ankle strength by having the patient push his foot down against your resistance and then pull his foot up as you try to hold it down.

Abnormal findings

Abnormalities in the musculoskeletal system occur for many reasons. Some general abnormalities have already been discussed; more specific ones are described below.

Rheumatoid arthritis

Rheumatoid arthritis is a chronic, systemic, inflammatory disease that attacks the joints and surrounding tissues, especially the hands, hips, knees, and feet. It causes loss of motion, symmetrical joint pain, joint tenderness, and stiffness or fixation of a joint, called ankylosis. The cause is unknown, although infectious, genetic, and endocrine factors may be responsible.

In this disorder, inflammation causes swelling, heat, and redness. Deformity appears first in the fingers and progresses to contractures. Crepitus is present.

Osteoarthritis

Osteoarthritis is the chronic degeneration of joint cartilage caused by aging or trauma. New bone forms at the joints. Symptoms vary from stiffness and mild aches to joint swelling, pain, deformity, crepitus, limitation of movement, and contracture. Gait may be affected if knees and hips are involved. Fingers may develop hard nodes on the distal and proximal joints. (See *Heberden's and Bouchard's nodes.*)

Gout

With gout, or gouty arthritis, urate crystals are deposited in joints, causing them to be red, swollen, and acutely painful. Irregular yellow-white bumps or nodules, called tophi, may develop on the great toe and the pinna of the ear from crystal deposits. Causes include renal disease and a family history of gout.

Heberden's and Bouchard's nodes

Heberden's and Bouchard's nodes are typically seen in patients with osteoarthritis.

Heberden's nodes
These nodes appear on the distal interphalangeal joints. Usually hard and painless, these bony and cartilaginous enlargements typically occur in middle-aged and elderly osteoarthritic patients.

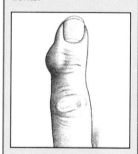

Bouchard's nodes
Bouchard's nodes are similar but less common and appear on the proximal interphalangeal joints.

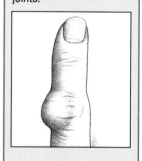

Tendinitis and bursitis

Caused by stress on a tendon or joint, tendinitis is the inflammation of the tendons and muscle attachments to bone, especially in the hip, shoulder, Achilles tendon, and elbow. Fluid may accumulate in the joint, causing swelling, limited movement, and pain.

Bursitis involves the bursae surrounding a joint and results from trauma or inflammatory joint disease. It causes pain and limited movement.

Osteoporosis

A decrease in bone mass, osteoporosis causes bones to become porous, brittle, and prone to fracture. A humped back, loss of height, and pain from a possible vertebral fracture are clues to osteoporosis. This condition is most common in postmenopausal women; other predisposing factors include prolonged immobility and low dietary intake of calcium.

Herniated disk

Most herniations occur in the lumbar spine. (See *Herniated disk*.) The patient's posture will be lateral and forward bending. He may also have unilateral low back pain radiating to the buttock, leg, and foot and sciatic pain or muscle spasms. Causes include spinal trauma, heavy lifting, lack of exercise, weight gain, and degenerative changes.

Rotator cuff injury

The rotator cuff — powerful muscles and tendons that surround the ball and socket of the shoulder — supports and stabilizes this joint. An injury to the rotator cuff causes shoulder pain, spasm, and limited range of motion. It also causes sudden dropping of the arm after the patient has abducted it. A rotator cuff injury may result from a fall on the shoulder or from activities like throwing and heavy lifting.

Carpal tunnel syndrome

Pain on wrist flexion and burning or tingling along the median nerve indicates carpal tunnel syndrome. It results from compression of the median nerve in the wrist as it passes through the carpal tunnel. Paresthesia may affect the thumb, forefinger, middle finger, and half of the ring finger.

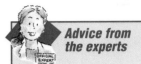

Advice from the experts

Herniated disk

If you suspect a herniated disk, perform the straight-leg-raising test. Have the patient lie supine. Ask him to raise one leg while keeping his knee extended, and then dorsiflex his foot. If this movement triggers sciatica — posterior leg pain — he probably has a herniated disk.

The 5 P's of musculoskeletal injury

To swiftly assess a musculoskeletal injury, remember the 5 P's — pain, paresthesia, paralysis, pallor, and pulse.

Pain

Ask the patient if he's having pain. If he is, assess the location, severity, and quality of the pain as well as anything that seems to relieve or worsen it.

Paresthesia

Assess for loss of sensation by touching the injured area with the tip of an open safety pin or the point of a paper clip. Then assess the same area on the unaffected side and compare. Abnormal sensation or loss of sensation indicates neurovascular involvement.

Paralysis

Can the patient move the affected area? If he can't, or if movement causes severe pain and muscle spasms, he might have nerve or tendon damage.

Pallor

Paleness, discoloration, and coolness on the injured side may indicate neurovascular compromise from decreased blood supply to the area.

Pulse

Check all pulses distal to the injury site. If a pulse is decreased or absent, blood supply to the area is reduced.

The causes are many, including sustained grasping, twisting, or flexing of the wrist; pregnancy; rheumatoid arthritis; diabetes mellitus; and dislocation or acute sprain of the wrist.

Musculoskeletal trauma

Most musculoskeletal emergencies result from trauma. Specific traumatic injuries include fractures, dislocations, amputations, crush injuries, and serious lacerations. The patient usually is alert and able to describe how the injury occurred.

If his level of consciousness deteriorates, suspect shock or drug or alcohol ingestion and assess further. (See *The 5 P's of musculoskeletal injury.*) *Remember, even if the patient has ingested drugs or alcohol, he can still go into shock.*

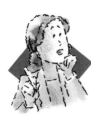

Quick quiz

1. If you hear crepitus while moving a patient's joint, the joint must be:

    A.   synovial.

    B.   nonsynovial.

    C.   fixed.

Answer: A. Crepitus occurs when roughened articular surfaces of bone or bone fragments rub together. So it can only occur in joints that are freely movable such as the synovial joints. Nonsynovial joints contain fused bones, so they don't move.

2. Rheumatoid arthritis is characterized by:

    A.   unilateral joint involvement.

    B.   nonsynovial joint involvement.

    C.   symmetrical joint involvement.

Answer: C. Rheumatoid arthritis produces symmetrical joint pain and loss of function.

3. If your patient's arm drifts down after he extends it for 10 seconds, he probably has:

    A.   carpal tunnel syndrome.

    B.   broken metatarsal bones.

    C.   shoulder-girdle weakness.

Answer: C. Inability to lift and extend an arm for 30 seconds indicates weakness of the shoulder girdle muscles on that side.

4. A patient with kyphosis has an:

    A.   exaggerated lateral spinal curvature.

    B.   unusually rounded thoracic curve.

    C.   abnormally concave lumbar spine.

Answer: B. Kyphosis causes a rounded back in the thoracic region.

5. Your patient can't move his right arm away from his side, so you document this as impaired:

    A.   supination.

    B.   abduction.

    C.   eversion.

Answer: B. Abduction is the ability to move a limb away from the midline.

6. To assess a swollen knee, perform the:
   A. bulge sign test.
   B. straight-leg-raising test
   C. dorsiflexion test.

Answer: A. A swollen knee suggests excess fluid in the joint. The bulge sign occurs when you apply pressure to the knee and a bulge of fluid appears on the opposite side.

Scoring

☆☆☆ If you answered all six items correctly, hip, hip, hooray! You've got big enough muscles to be a bouncer at the Synovial Joint!

☆☆ If you answered four or five items correctly, yeah! You're by far the best dancer at Club Ball-N-Socket!

☆ If you answered fewer than four items correctly, that's okay! You're the up-and-comer at the Hip-Hop Hinge Joint!

Neurologic system

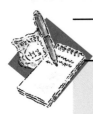

Just the facts

This chapter discusses the neurologic system. In this chapter, you'll learn:

♦ how to identify organs and structures that make up the neurologic system

♦ how to obtain information about neurologic function from the patient history

♦ how to conduct a physical assessment of the neurologic system

♦ how to recognize neurologic abnormalities.

A look at the neurologic system

The neurologic system controls body function and is related to every other body system. Consequently, patients who suffer from diseases of other body systems can develop neurologic impairments related to the disease. One example of this is a patient who has heart surgery and then suffers a cerebrovascular accident.

Because the neurologic system is so complex, evaluating it can seem overwhelming at first. Although tests for neurologic status are extensive, they're also basic and straightforward. In fact, your daily nursing care may routinely include some of these tests.

Just talking with a patient helps you assess his orientation, level of consciousness (LOC), and ability to formulate and produce speech. Having him perform a simple task such as walking allows you to evaluate motor ability. Your knowledge of neurologic anatomy, physiology, and assessment techniques will enhance your patient care and may save some patients from irreversible neurologic damage.

Three-part system

The neurologic system is divided into the central nervous system, the peripheral nervous system, and the autonomic nervous system. Through complex and coordinated interactions, these three parts integrate all physical, intellectual, and emotional activities. Understanding how these three parts work is essential to conducting an accurate neurologic assessment.

Central nervous system

The central nervous system includes the brain and the spinal cord. (See *A close look at the central nervous system.*) These two structures collect and interpret voluntary and involuntary motor and sensory stimuli.

A close look at the central nervous system

This illustration shows a cross section of the brain and spinal cord, which together make up the central nervous system. The brain joins the spinal cord at the base of the skull and ends near the second lumbar vertebrae. Note the H-shaped mass of gray matter in the spinal cord.

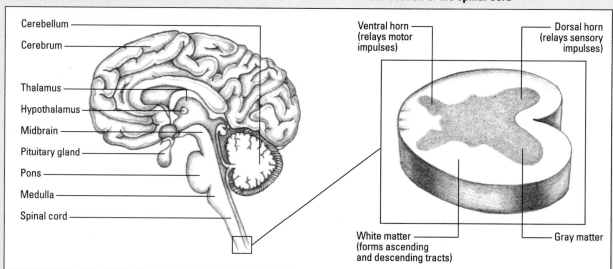

Cross section of the brain

- Cerebellum
- Cerebrum
- Thalamus
- Hypothalamus
- Midbrain
- Pituitary gland
- Pons
- Medulla
- Spinal cord

Cross section of the spinal cord

- Ventral horn (relays motor impulses)
- Dorsal horn (relays sensory impulses)
- White matter (forms ascending and descending tracts)
- Gray matter

Brain

The brain consists of the cerebrum or cerebral cortex, the brain stem, and the cerebellum. It collects, integrates, and interprets all stimuli and initiates and monitors voluntary and involuntary motor activity.

The reason for your cerebrum

The cerebrum gives us the ability to think and reason. It's encased by the skull and enclosed by three membrane layers called meninges. If blood or fluid accumulates between these layers, pressure builds inside the skull and compromises brain function.

The cerebrum is divided into four lobes and two hemispheres. The right hemisphere controls the left side of the body, and the left hemisphere controls the right side of the body. Each lobe controls different functions. (See *A close look at the cerebrum and its functions.*)

A close look at the cerebrum and its functions

The cerebrum is divided into four lobes based on anatomic landmarks and functional differences. The lobes — parietal, occipital, temporal, and frontal — are named for the cranial bones that lie over them.

The illustration shows the locations of the cerebral lobes and explains their functions. It also shows the location of the cerebellum.

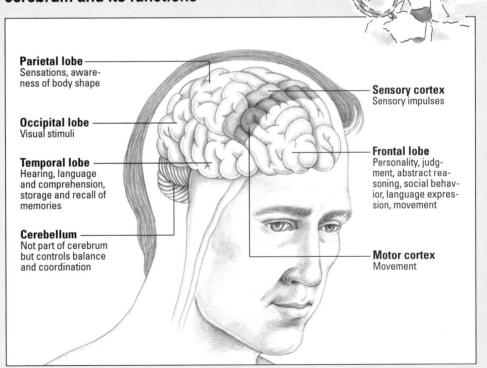

Parietal lobe
Sensations, awareness of body shape

Occipital lobe
Visual stimuli

Temporal lobe
Hearing, language and comprehension, storage and recall of memories

Cerebellum
Not part of cerebrum but controls balance and coordination

Sensory cortex
Sensory impulses

Frontal lobe
Personality, judgment, abstract reasoning, social behavior, language expression, movement

Motor cortex
Movement

Meet the muses, Thala and Hypothala

The diencephalon, a division of the cerebrum, contains the thalamus and hypothalamus. The thalamus is a relay station for sensory impulses. The hypothalamus has many regulatory functions, including temperature control, pituitary hormone production, and water balance.

A stem with three parts

The brain stem lies below the diencephalon and is divided into the midbrain, pons, and medulla. The brain stem contains the nuclei of cranial nerves III through XII and is a major sensory and motor pathway for impulses running to and from the cerebral cortex. It also regulates automatic body functions like heart rate, breathing, swallowing, and coughing.

Go to the back of the brain

The cerebellum, the most posterior part of the brain, contains the major motor and sensory pathways. It facilitates smooth, coordinated muscle movement and helps to maintain equilibrium.

Spinal cord

The spinal cord is the primary pathway for messages traveling between the peripheral areas of the body and the brain. It also mediates the sensory-to-motor transmission path known as the reflex arc. (See *Reflex arc.*) Because the reflex arc enters and exits the spinal cord at the same level, reflex pathways don't need to travel up and down the way other stimuli do.

The spinal cord extends from the upper border of the first cervical vertebrae to the lower border of the first lumbar vertebrae. It's encased by the same membrane structure as the brain and is protected by the bony vertebrae of the spine.

The dorsal white matter contains the ascending tracts that carry impulses up the spinal cord to higher sensory centers. The ventral white matter contains the descending motor tracts that transmit motor impulses down from the higher motor centers to the spinal cord.

Mapping out the body

For the purpose of documenting sensory function, the body is divided into dermatomes. Each dermatome repre-

Reflex arc

Spinal nerves, which have sensory and motor portions, control deep tendon and superficial reflexes. A simple reflex arc requires a sensory or afferent neuron and a motor or efferent neuron. The knee-jerk or patellar reflex illustrates the sequence of events in a normal reflex arc.

First, a sensory receptor detects the mechanical stimulus produced by the reflex hammer striking the patellar tendon. Then the sensory neuron carries the impulse along its axon by way of a spinal nerve to the dorsal root, where it enters the spinal column.

Next, in the anterior horn of the spinal cord, shown here, the sensory neuron joins with a motor neuron, which carries the impulse along its axon by way of a spinal nerve to the muscle. The motor neuron transmits the impulse to the muscle fibers through stimulation of the motor end plate. This triggers the muscle to contract and the leg to extend. *Don't stand directly in front of a patient when testing this reflex!*

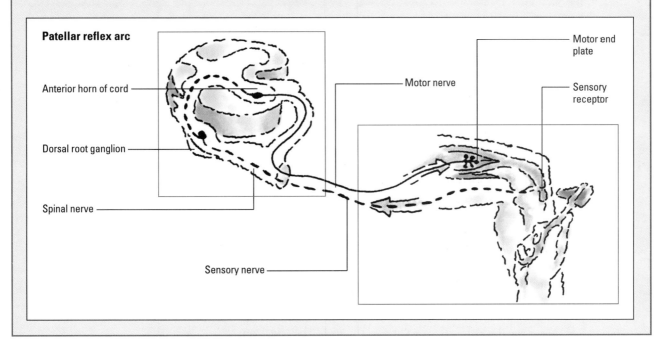

Patellar reflex arc

Anterior horn of cord

Dorsal root ganglion

Spinal nerve

Sensory nerve

Motor nerve

Motor end plate

Sensory receptor

sents an area supplied with afferent, or sensory, nerve fibers from an individual spinal root — either cervical, thoracic, lumbar, or sacral. This body "map" is used when testing sensation and trying to identify the source of a lesion.

Peripheral nervous system

The peripheral nervous system includes the peripheral and cranial nerves. Peripheral sensory nerves transmit stimuli to the dorsal horn of the spinal cord from sensory

Identifying cranial nerves

The cranial nerves have either sensory or motor function or both. They're assigned Roman numerals and are written this way: CN I, CN II, CN III, and so forth. The illustration shows the functions of the cranial nerves.

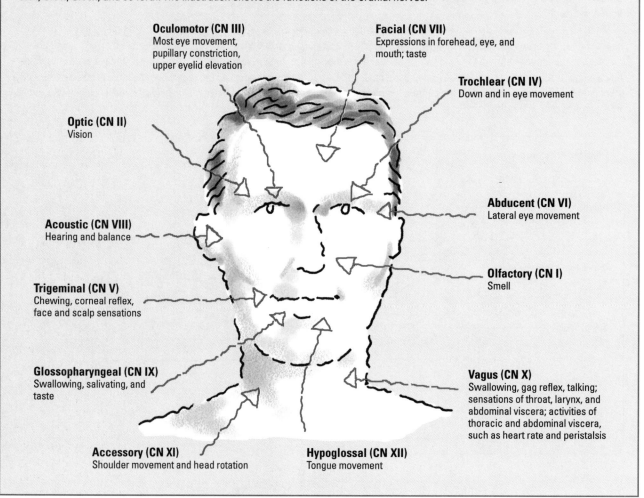

Oculomotor (CN III)
Most eye movement, pupillary constriction, upper eyelid elevation

Facial (CN VII)
Expressions in forehead, eye, and mouth; taste

Trochlear (CN IV)
Down and in eye movement

Optic (CN II)
Vision

Abducent (CN VI)
Lateral eye movement

Acoustic (CN VIII)
Hearing and balance

Olfactory (CN I)
Smell

Trigeminal (CN V)
Chewing, corneal reflex, face and scalp sensations

Glossopharyngeal (CN IX)
Swallowing, salivating, and taste

Vagus (CN X)
Swallowing, gag reflex, talking; sensations of throat, larynx, and abdominal viscera; activities of thoracic and abdominal viscera, such as heart rate and peristalsis

Accessory (CN XI)
Shoulder movement and head rotation

Hypoglossal (CN XII)
Tongue movement

receptors located in the skin, muscles, sensory organs, and viscera. The upper motor neurons of the brain and the lower motor neurons of the cell bodies in the ventral horn of the spinal cord carry impulses that affect movement.

The 12 pairs of cranial nerves are the primary motor and sensory pathways between the brain, head, and neck. (See *Identifying cranial nerves*.)

Autonomic nervous system

The autonomic nervous system contains motor neurons that regulate the activities of the visceral organs and affect the smooth and cardiac muscles and the glands. It consists of two parts: the sympathetic division, which controls fight or flight reactions, and the parasympathetic division, which maintains baseline body functions.

Obtaining a health history

The most common chief complaints about the neurologic system include headache, dizziness, faintness, confusion, impaired mental status, disturbances in balance or gait, and changes in LOC. When documenting the chief complaint, record the information in the patient's own words.

So, fill me in on the details

Once you learn the chief complaint, ask the patient about its onset and frequency, what precipitates or exacerbates it, and what alleviates it. Ask if other symptoms accompany the chief complaint and if he has had adverse effects from treatments.

Also ask about other aspects of his current health and about his past health and family history. Help him describe problems by asking pertinent questions like those below.

Asking about current health

Ask the patient if he has headaches. If so, how often, when, and what seems to bring them on? Does light bother his eyes during a headache? What other symptoms occur with the headache?

Does the patient have dizziness, numbness, tingling, seizures, tremors, weakness, or paralysis? Does he have problems with any of his senses or with walking, keeping his balance, swallowing, or urinating?

How does he rate his memory and ability to concentrate? Does he ever have trouble speaking or understanding people? Does he have trouble reading or writing? If he has these problems, how much do they interfere with his daily activities?

Keep in mind that some neurologic changes, such as decreased reflexes, hearing, and vision, are a normal part of aging. (See *Aging and the neurologic system*.)

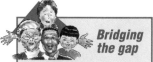

Bridging the gap

Aging and the neurologic system

Because neurons undergo various degenerative changes, aging can lead to:

- diminished reflexes
- decreased hearing, vision, taste, and smell
- slowed reaction time
- decreased agility
- decreased vibratory sense in the ankles
- development of muscles tremors, such as in the head and hands

Look beyond age
Remember that not all neurologic changes in the elderly are caused by aging. Certain medications can cause neurologic changes as well. Check to see if the changes are asymmetric, indicating a pathologic condition, or if other abnormalities in the neurologic examination need further investigation.

Asking about past health

Because many chronic diseases can affect the neurologic system, ask the patient about his past health. Inquire about major illnesses, recurrent minor illnesses, accidents or injuries, surgical procedures, and allergies. Don't forget to ask what medications he's taking, since many medications can affect the neurologic system.

Asking about family history

Finally, ask about his family history. Some genetic diseases are degenerative; others cause muscle weakness. For example, the incidence of seizures is higher in patients whose family history shows idiopathic epilepsy, and more than half of patients with migraine headaches have a family history of the disorder.

Assessing the neurologic system

A complete neurologic examination is so long and detailed that you probably won't ever perform one in its entirety. However, if your initial screening examination suggests a neurologic problem, you may want to perform a more detailed assessment.

Always examine the patient's neurologic system in an orderly fashion. Begin with the highest levels of neurologic function and work down to the lowest, covering these five areas:
- mental status and speech
- cranial nerve function
- sensory function
- motor function
- reflexes.

Assessing mental status and speech

Your mental status assessment actually begins when you talk to the patient during the health history. How he responds to your questions gives clues to his orientation and memory and guides you during your physical assessment.

Be sure to ask questions that require more than a yes-or-no answer. Otherwise, confusion or disorientation might not be immediately apparent. If you have doubts about a patient's mental status, perform a screening examination. (See *A quick check of mental status*.)

Another guide during the physical assessment is the patient's history and chief complaint. For example, if he complains about confusion or memory problems, you'll want to concentrate on the mental status part of the examination.

Stop, look, and listen

The mental status examination consists of checking LOC, appearance, behavior, speech, cognitive function, and constructional ability.

Level of consciousness

A change in the patient's LOC is the earliest and most sensitive indicator that his neurologic status has changed.

Peak technique

A quick check of mental status

To quickly screen patients for disordered thought processes, ask the questions below. An incorrect answer to any question may indicate the need for a complete mental status examination. Make sure you know the correct answers before asking the questions.

Question	Function screened
What is your name?	Orientation to person
What is your mother's name?	Orientation to other people
What is today's date?	Orientation to time
What year is it?	Orientation to time
Where are you now?	Orientation to place
How old are you?	Memory
Where were you born?	Remote memory
What did you have for breakfast?	Recent memory
Why are you here?	Recent memory
Who is the U.S. president?	General knowledge
Can you count backward from 20 to 1?	Attention span and calculation skills
Can you repeat the numbers 2, 8, 11, 14, 20?	Attention span and calculation skills

Many terms are used to describe LOC, but their definitions may differ slightly among practitioners. To avoid confusion, clearly describe the patient's response to various stimuli using these guidelines:

• alert — follows commands and responds completely and appropriately to stimuli

• lethargic — drowsy, delayed responses to verbal stimuli, may drift off to sleep during examination

• stuporous — requires vigorous stimulation for a response

• comatose — doesn't respond appropriately to verbal or painful stimuli, can't follow commands or communicate verbally.

Perky or drowsy?

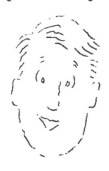

During your assessment, observe the patient's LOC. Is he alert or falling asleep? Can he focus his attention and maintain it, or is he easily distracted? If you need to use a stronger stimulus than your voice, record what it is and how strong it needs to be to get a response from the patient. The Glasgow Coma Scale offers a more objective way to assess the patient's LOC. (See *Glasgow Coma Scale.*)

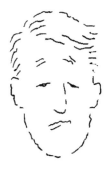

Appearance and behavior

Also note how the patient behaves, dresses, and grooms himself. Does he look and act inappropriately? Is his personal hygiene poor? If so, discuss your findings with the family to determine if this is a change. *Even subtle changes in a patient's behavior can signal a new onset of a chronic disease or a more acute change that involves the frontal lobe.*

Speech

Next, listen to how well the patient can express himself. Is his speech fluent or fragmented? Note the pace, volume, clarity, and spontaneity of his speech. To assess for dysarthria, or difficulty forming words, ask him to repeat the phrase "No ifs, ands, or buts." Assess comprehension by determining his ability to follow instructions and cooperate with your examination.

Cognitive function

Assessing cognitive function involves testing the patient's memory, orientation, attention span, calculation ability,

What does it all mean?

Glasgow Coma Scale

The Glasgow Coma Scale provides an easy way to describe the patient's baseline mental status and to help detect and interpret changes from baseline findings. To use the Glasgow Coma Scale, test the patient's ability to respond to verbal, motor, and sensory stimulation and grade your findings according to the scale. If a patient is alert, can follow simple commands, and is oriented to person, place, and time, his score will total 15 points. A decreased score in one or more categories may signal an impending neurologic crisis. A total score of 7 or less indicates severe neurologic damage.

Test	Score	Patient's response
Eye opening response		
Spontaneously	4	Opens eyes spontaneously
To speech	3	Opens eyes when told to
To pain	2	Opens eyes only on painful stimulus
None	1	Doesn't open eyes in response to stimulus
Motor response		
Obeys	6	Shows two fingers when asked
Localizes	5	Reaches toward painful stimulus and tries to remove it
Withdraws	4	Moves away from painful stimulus
Abnormal flexion	3	Assumes a decorticate posture (below)
Abnormal extension	2	Assumes a decerebrate posture (below)
None	1	No response; just lies flaccid — an ominous sign
Verbal response to question, "What year is this?"		
Oriented	5	Tells current date
Confused	4	Tells incorrect year
Inappropriate words	3	Replies randomly with incorrect word
Incomprehensible	2	Moans or screams
None	1	No response
Total score		

thought content, abstract thinking, judgment, insight, and emotional status.

Telltale testing

To quickly test your patient's orientation, memory, and attention span, use the mental status screening questions discussed previously. Orientation to time is usually disrupted first; orientation to person, last.

Always consider the patient's environment and physical condition when assessing orientation. For example, an elderly patient admitted to the hospital for several days may not be oriented to time, especially if he's been bedridden. Also, when the person is intubated and unable to speak, ask questions that require only a nod: "Do you know you're in the hospital?" "Are we in Pennsylvania?"

The patient with an intact short-term memory can generally repeat five to seven nonconsecutive numbers right away and again 10 minutes later. *Remember that short-term memory is often affected first in neurologic disease.*

When testing attention span and calculation skills, keep in mind that lack of mathematical ability and anxiety can affect the patient's performance. If he has difficulty with numerical computation, ask him to spell the word "world" backwards. While he's performing these functions, note his ability to pay attention.

Clear and cogent?

Assess thought content by evaluating the clarity and cohesiveness of the patient's ideas. Is his conversation smooth, with logical transitions between ideas? Does he have hallucinations — sensory perceptions that lack appropriate stimuli — or delusions — beliefs not supported by reality? Disordered thought patterns may indicate delirium or psychosis.

The proverbial abstract-thinking test

Test the patient's ability to think abstractly by asking him to interpret a common proverb such as "a stitch in time saves nine." A person with dementia may interpret this proverb literally. If the patient's primary language isn't English, he will normally have difficulty interpreting the proverb. Engage the assistance of family members when English is not the patient's primary language. Have them ask the patient to explain a saying in his native language.

What if...?

Test the patient's judgment by asking him how he would respond to a hypothetical situation. For example, what would he do if he were in a public building and the fire alarm sounded? Evaluate the appropriateness of his answer.

Feelings, nothing more than feelings

Throughout the interview, assess the patient's emotional status. Note his mood, his emotional lability or stability, and the appropriateness of his emotional responses. Also assess his mood by asking how he feels about himself and his future. *Keep in mind that symptoms of depression in elderly patients may be atypical — for example, decreased function or increased agitation rather than the usual sad affect.*

Constructional ability

Constructional disorders affect the patient's ability to perform simple tasks and use various objects.

Assessing cranial nerve function

There are twelve pairs of cranial nerves. These nerves transmit motor or sensory messages, or both, primarily between the brain and brain stem and the head and neck.

The sense of smell

Assess cranial nerve I, the olfactory nerve, first. Make sure the patient's nostrils are patent. Have him identify at least two common substances, such as coffee, cinnamon, or cloves. Avoid stringent odors, such as ammonia or peppermint, which stimulate the trigeminal nerve.

Seeing eye to eye

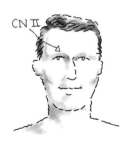

CN II

Next, assess cranial nerve II, the optic nerve. To test visual acuity quickly and informally, have the patient read a newspaper, starting with large headlines and moving to small print.

Test visual fields with a technique called confrontation. To do this, stand 2′ (0.6 m) in front of the patient, and have him cover one eye. Then close one of your eyes and bring your moving fingers into the patient's visual field from the periphery. Ask him to tell you when he sees the object. Test each quadrant of the patient's visual field, and

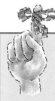

Memory jogger

To help you remember cranial nerve order, think of the mnemonic you learned in school: "On Old Olympus' Towering Tops, A Finn And German Viewed Some Hops." The first letter of each word stands for the first letter in cranial nerves I through XII.

Olfactory (CN I)
Optic (CN II)
Oculomotor (CN III)
Trochlear (CN IV)
Trigeminal (CN V)
Abducens (CN VI)
Facial (CN VII)
Acoustic (CN VIII)
Glossopharyngeal (CN IX)
Vagus (CN X)
Spinal accessory (CN XI)
Hypoglossal (CN XII)

compare his results with your own. Chart any defects you find. (See *Visual field defects*.)

Finally, examine the fundus of the optic nerve, as described in Chapter 5. Blurring of the optic disc may indicate increased intracranial pressure.

Three real lookers

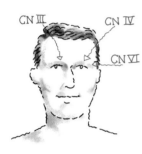

The oculomotor nerve (cranial nerve III), the trochlear nerve (cranial nerve IV), and the abducent nerve (cranial nerve VI) all control eye movement. So assess these nerves together.

The oculomotor nerve controls most extraocular movement; it's also responsible for elevation of the eyelid and pupillary constriction. Abnormalities include ptosis, or drooping of the upper lid, and pupil inequality. Make sure the patient's pupils constrict when exposed to light and his eyes accommodate for seeing objects at various distances.

Also, ask the patient to follow your finger through the six cardinal positions of gaze:
1. left superior
2. left lateral
3. left inferior
4. right superior
5. right lateral
6. right inferior

Pause slightly before moving from one position to the next to assess for nystagmus, or involuntary eye movement, and the ability to hold the gaze in that particular position.

Tri chewing without this nerve

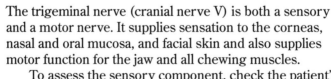

The trigeminal nerve (cranial nerve V) is both a sensory and a motor nerve. It supplies sensation to the corneas, nasal and oral mucosa, and facial skin and also supplies motor function for the jaw and all chewing muscles.

To assess the sensory component, check the patient's ability to feel light touch on his face. Ask him to close his eyes; then touch him with a wisp of cotton on his forehead, cheek, and jaw on each side. Next, test pain perception by touching the tip of a safety pin to the same three areas. Ask the patient to describe and compare both sensations.

Alternate the touches between sharp and dull to test the patient's reliability in comparing sensations. Proper as-

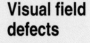

Visual field defects

Here are some examples of visual field defects. The black areas represent visual loss.

Left	Right

A: Blindness of right eye

B: Bitemporal hemianopia, or loss of half the visual field

C: Left homonymous hemianopia

D: Left homonymous hemianopia, superior quadrant

sessment of the nerve requires that the patient identify sharp stimuli. To test the motor component of cranial nerve V, ask the patient to clench his teeth while you palpate the temporal and masseter muscles.

Taking a taste test

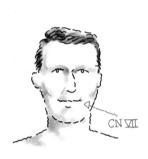

The facial nerve (cranial nerve VII) also has both a sensory and motor component. The sensory component controls taste perception on the anterior part of the tongue. It can be assessed by asking the patient to taste sweet, sour, salty, and bitter substances; however, this isn't usually done. If you do attempt it, have the patient follow each taste with a sip of water.

The motor component is responsible for the facial muscles. Assess this by observing the patient's face for symmetry at rest and while he smiles, frowns, and raises his eyebrows.

If a weakness is caused by a stroke or other condition that damages the cortex, the patient will be able to raise his eyebrows and wrinkle his forehead. If the weakness is due to an interruption of the facial nerve or other peripheral nerve involvement, the entire side of his face will be immobile.

Let's hear it for the acoustic nerve!

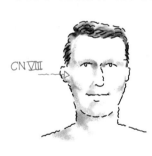

The acoustic nerve (cranial nerve VIII) is responsible for hearing and equilibrium. The cochlear division controls hearing, and the vestibular division controls balance.

To test hearing, ask the patient to cover one ear, and then stand on his opposite side and whisper a few words. See if he can repeat what you said. Test the other ear the same way.

To test the vestibular portion of this nerve, observe for nystagmus and disturbed balance, and note reports of dizziness or the room spinning.

Not so hard to swallow

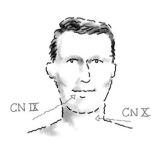

The glossopharyngeal nerve (cranial nerve IX) and the vagus nerve (cranial nerve X) are tested together because their innervation overlaps in the pharynx. The glossopharyngeal nerve is responsible for swallowing, salivating, and taste perception on the posterior one-third of the tongue. The vagus nerve controls swallowing and is also responsible for voice quality.

Start your assessment by listening to the patient's voice. Then check his gag reflex by touching the tip of a tongue blade against his posterior pharynx and asking him to open wide and say "ah." Observe for the symmetrical upward movement of the soft palate and uvula and for the midline position of the uvula.

A very important accessory

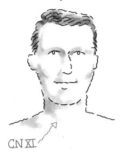

CN XI

A motor nerve, the spinal accessory nerve (cranial nerve XI) controls the sternocleidomastoid muscles and the upper portion of the trapezius muscles. To assess this nerve, test the strength of both muscles. First, place your palm against the patient's cheek; then ask him to turn his head against your resistance.

Test the trapezius muscle by placing your hands on the patient's shoulder and asking him to shrug his shoulders against your resistance. Repeat each test on the other side, comparing muscle strength.

Speaking about the tongue

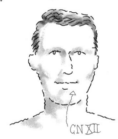

CN XII

The hypoglossal nerve (cranial nerve XII) controls tongue movement involved in swallowing and speech. The tongue should be midline, without tremors or fasciculations. Test tongue strength by asking the patient to push his tongue against his cheek as you offer resistance. Observe his tongue for symmetry. Test his speech by asking him to repeat the sentence "Round the rugged rock the ragged rascal ran."

Assessing sensory function

Evaluation of the sensory system involves checking these five areas of sensation: pain, light touch, vibration, position, and discrimination.

This may hurt a bit

To test the patient for pain sensation, have him close his eyes; then touch all the major dermatomes first with the sharp end of a safety pin and then with the dull end. Proceed in this order: fingers, shoulders, toes, thighs, and trunk. Ask him to identify when he feels the sharp stimulus.

If the patient has major deficits, start in the area with the least sensation and move toward the area with the most sensation. This helps you determine the level of deficit.

Getting in touch

To test for the sense of light touch, follow the same routine as above, but use a wisp of cotton. Lightly touch the patient's skin — don't swab or sweep the cotton because you might miss an area of loss. A patient with a peripheral neuropathy might retain his sensation for light touch after he's lost pain sensation.

Good vibrations

To test vibratory sense, apply a tuning fork over certain bony prominences while the patient keeps his eyes closed. (See *Evaluating vibratory sense*.) Start at the distal interphalangeal joint of the index finger and move proximally. Test only until the patient feels the vibration because everything above that level will be intact.

If vibratory sense is intact, you won't have to check position sense because the same pathway carries both.

Fingers and toes on the move

To assess position sense, have the patient close his eyes. Then grasp the sides of his big toe, move it up and down, and ask him what position it's in. To be tested for position sense, the patient needs intact vestibular and cerebellar function.

Perform the same test on the patient's upper extremities by grasping the sides of his index finger and moving it back and forth.

Rate ability to discriminate

Discriminatory testing assesses the ability of the cerebral cortex to interpret and integrate information. Stereognosis is the ability to discriminate the shape, size, weight, texture, and form of an object by touching and manipulating it. To test this, ask the patient to close his eyes and open his hand. Then place a common object such as a key in his hand, and ask him to identify it.

If he can't, test graphesthesia next. Have the patient keep his eyes closed and hold out his hand while you draw a large number on the palm. Ask him to identify the number. Both these tests assess the ability of the cortex to integrate sensory input.

To test point localization, have the patient close his eyes; then touch one of his limbs and ask him where you touched him. Test two point discrimination by touching the patient simultaneously in two contralateral areas. He should be able to identify both touches. Failure to perceive touch on one side is called extinction.

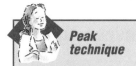

Peak technique

Evaluating vibratory sense

To evaluate vibratory sense, apply the base of a vibrating tuning fork to the interphalangeal joint of the patient's great toe, as shown below. Ask him what he feels. If he feels the sensation, he'll typically report a feeling of buzzing or vibration.

If he doesn't feel the vibration at the toe, try the medial malleolus. Then continue moving proximally until he feels the vibration. Note where he feels it, and then repeat the process on the other leg.

Assessing motor function

Assessing the motor system includes inspecting the muscles and testing muscle tone and muscle strength. Cerebellar testing is also done because the cerebellum plays a role in smooth muscle movements, balance, and gait.

First inspect muscle size, contour, and symmetry. Then observe for abnormal movements, such as tics, tremors, or fasciculation.

Muscle tone

Muscle tone represents muscular resistance to passive stretching. To test arm muscle tone, move the patient's shoulder through passive range-of-motion exercises. You should feel a slight resistance. Then let the arm drop to the patient's side. It should fall easily.

To test leg muscle tone, guide the hip through passive range-of-motion exercises; then let the leg fall to the bed. If it falls into an externally rotated position, this is an abnormal finding.

Muscle strength

A general examination of muscle strength can be done by observing the patient's gait and motor activities. To evaluate muscle strength, ask the patient to move major muscles and muscle groups against resistance. For instance, to test shoulder girdle strength, have him extend his arms with his palms up and maintain this position for 30 seconds.

If he can't maintain this position, test further by pushing down on his outstretched arms. If he does lift both arms equally, look for pronation of the hand and downward drift of the arm on the weaker side.

Cerebellum

Cerebellar testing looks at the patient's coordination and general balance. Can he sit and stand without support? If so, observe him as he walks across the room, turns, and walks back. Note imbalances or abnormalities.

With cerebellar dysfunction, the patient will have a wide-based, unsteady gait. Deviation to one side may indicate a cerebellar lesion on that side. Ask the patient to

Romberg's test

Observe the patient's balance as he stands with his eyes open, feet together, and arms at his side. Then ask him to close his eyes. Hold your arms out on either side of him to protect him if he sways. If he falls to one side, Romberg's test is positive.

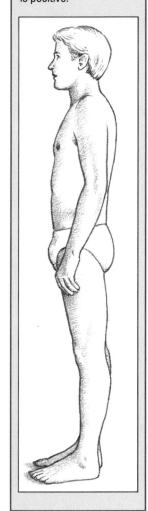

walk heel to toe and observe his balance. Then perform Romberg's test. (See *Romberg's test.*)

Nose-to-finger test

Test extremity coordination by asking the patient to touch his nose and then touch your outstretched finger as you move it. Have him do this faster and faster. His movements should be accurate and smooth.

Quick, do these tests!

Other tests of cerebellar function assess rapid alternating movements. In these tests, the patient's movements should be accurate and smooth.

First ask the patient to touch the thumb of his right hand to his right index finger and then to each of his remaining fingers. Observe the movements for accuracy and smoothness. Next ask him to sit with his palms on his thighs. Tell him to turn his palms up and down, gradually increasing his speed.

Sole tapping

Finally, have the patient lie supine. Then stand at the foot of the table or bed and hold your palms near his soles. Ask him to alternately tap the sole of his right foot and the sole of his left foot against your palms. He should increase his speed as you observe his coordination.

Assessing reflexes

Evaluating reflexes involves testing deep tendon reflexes and superficial reflexes and observing for primitive reflexes.

Deep tendon reflexes

The key to testing deep tendon reflexes is to make sure the patient is relaxed and the joint is flexed appropriately. (See *Assessing deep tendon reflexes*, page 296.) First, distract the patient by asking him to focus on a point across the room. Always test deep tendon reflexes by moving from head to toe and comparing side to side.

Peak technique

Assessing deep tendon reflexes

During a neurologic examination, you'll assess the patient's deep tendon reflexes. Test the biceps, triceps, brachioradialis, patellar or quadriceps, and achilles reflexes.

Biceps reflex
Position the patient's arm so his elbow is flexed at a 45-degree angle and his arm is relaxed. Place your thumb or index finger over the biceps tendon and your remaining fingers loosely over the triceps muscle. Strike your finger with the pointed end of the reflex hammer, and watch and feel for the contraction of the biceps muscle and flexion of the forearm.

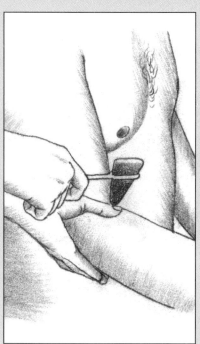

Triceps reflex
Have the patient abduct his arm and place his forearm across his chest. Strike the triceps tendon about 2″ (5 cm) above the olecranon process on the extensor surface of the upper arm. Watch for contraction of the triceps muscle and extension of the forearm.

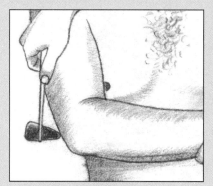

Brachioradialis reflex
Ask the patient to rest the ulnar surface of his hand on his knee with the elbow partially flexed. Strike the radius, and watch for supination of the hand and flexion of the forearm at the elbow.

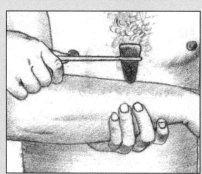

Patellar reflex
Have the patient sit with his legs dangling freely. If he can't sit up, flex his knee at a 45-degree angle, and place your nondominant hand behind it for support. Strike the patellar tendon just below the patella, and look for contraction of the quadriceps muscle in the thigh with extension of the leg.

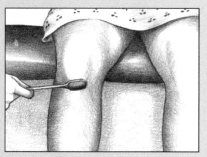

Achilles reflex
Have the patient flex his foot. Then support the plantar surface. Strike the achilles tendon, and watch for plantar flexion of the foot at the ankle.

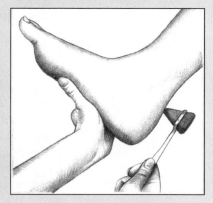

Grade deep tendon reflexes using the following scale:
 0 — absent impulses
+1 — diminished impulses
+2 — normal impulses
+3 — increased impulses but may be normal
+4 — hyperactive impulses.

Superficial reflexes

Superficial reflexes are tested by stimulating the skin or mucous membranes. *Because these are cutaneous reflexes, the more you try to elicit them in succession, the less of a response you'll get. So observe carefully the first time you stimulate.*

Tickling the feet

Using an applicator stick, tongue blade, or key, slowly stroke the lateral side of the patient's sole from the heel to the great toe. The normal response in an adult is plantar flexion of the toes. Upward movement of the great toe and fanning of the little toes — called Babinski's response — is normal in children under age 2 and abnormal in everyone else.

For men only

The cremasteric reflex is tested in men by using an applicator stick to stimulate the inner thigh. Normal reaction is contraction of the cremaster muscle and elevation of the testicle on the side of the stimulus.

Tickling the tummy

Test the abdominal reflexes with the patient in the supine position with his arms at his sides and his knees slightly flexed. Briskly stroke both sides of the abdomen above and below the umbilicus, moving from the periphery toward the midline. Movement of the umbilicus toward the stimulus is normal.

Primitive reflexes

Primitive reflexes are abnormal in adults but normal in infants, whose central nervous systems are immature. As the neurologic system matures, these reflexes disappear. The primitive reflexes you'll assess for are the grasp, snout, sucking, and glabella reflexes.

Just gotta grasp

Assess the grasp reflex by applying gentle pressure to the patient's palm with your fingers. If he grasps your fingers between his thumb and index finger, suspect cortical or premotor cortex damage.

Read my lip

The snout reflex is assessed by lightly tapping on the patient's upper lip. If the lip purses, this is a positive snout reflex indicating frontal lobe damage.

The urge to suck

Observe the patient while you're feeding him or if he has an oral airway or endotracheal tube in place. If you see a sucking motion, this indicates cortical damage. It's often seen in advanced dementia.

Tap, tap, blink, blink

The glabella response is elicited by repeatedly tapping the bridge of the patient's nose. The abnormal response is persistent blinking, which indicates diffuse cortical dysfunction.

Abnormal findings

During your assessment, you may detect abnormalities caused by neurologic dysfunction. The most common categories of abnormalities include altered LOC, cranial nerve impairment, abnormal muscle movements, and abnormal gaits.

Altered level of consciousness

Consciousness may be impaired by several disorders that affect the cerebral hemisphere or the brain stem. Consciousness is the most sensitive indicator of neurologic dysfunction and may be a valuable adjunct to other findings. (See *Detecting increased intracranial pressure*.) When assessing LOC, make sure that you provide a stimulus that's strong enough to get a true picture of the patient's baseline.

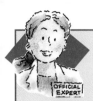

Advice from the experts

Detecting increased intracranial pressure

The earlier you can recognize the signs of increased intracranial pressure, the more quickly you can intervene and the better the patient's chance of recovery. By the time late signs appear, interventions may be useless.

	Early signs	Late signs
Level of consciousness	• Requires increased stimulation • Subtle orientation loss • Restlessness and anxiety • Sudden quietness	• Unarousable
Pupils	• Pupil changes on side of lesion • One pupil constricts but then dilates (unilateral hippus) • Sluggish reaction of both pupils • Unequal pupils	• Pupils fixed and dilated or "blown"
Motor response	• Sudden weakness • Motor changes on side opposite the lesion • Positive pronator drift; with palms up, one hand pronates	• Profound weakness
Vital signs	• Intermittent increases in blood pressure	• Increased systolic pressure, profound bradycardia, abnormal respirations (Cushing's syndrome)

Consciousness-altering disorders

Disorders that affect LOC include toxic encephalopathy, hemorrhage, and extensive, generalized cortical atrophy. Compression of brain-stem structures by tumor or hemorrhage also can affect consciousness by depressing the reticular activating system that maintains wakefulness. In addition, sedatives and narcotics can depress LOC.

Cranial nerve impairment

Damage to the cranial nerves causes many abnormalities including olfactory, visual, auditory, and muscular problems. Vertigo and dysphagia also can indicate cranial nerve damage.

Olfactory impairment

If the patient can't detect odors with both nostrils, he may have a dysfunction of cranial nerve I. This can result from any disease that affects the olfactory tract, such as a tumor, hemorrhage or, more commonly, a facial bone fracture that crosses the cribriform plate (portion of the ethmoid bone that separates the roof of the nose from the cranial cavity).

Visual impairment

Visual problems include visual field defects, pupillary changes, eye muscle impairment, and facial nerve impairment.

Visual field defects

Visual fields are affected by tumors or infarcts of the optic nerve head, optic chiasm, or optic tracts.

Pupillary changes

If the patient's pupillary response to light is affected, he may have damage to both the optic nerve and oculomotor nerve. (See *Understanding pupillary changes*.) Pupils are also sensitive indicators of neurologic demise. Increased intracranial pressure causes dilation of the pupil ipsilateral to the mass lesion but, without treatment, both pupils become fixed and dilated.

Anisocoria, or unequal pupils, is normal in about 20% of people. In normal anisocoria, pupil size doesn't change with the amount of illumination.

Eye muscle impairment

Weakness or paralysis of the eye muscles can result from cranial nerve damage. Increased intracranial pressure and intracranial lesions can affect the motor nuclei of the oculomotor, trochlear, and abducent nerves.

Nystagmus

Nystagmus can be caused by damage to the peripheral labyrinth, brain stem, or cerebellum. The eyes drift slowly in one direction and then jerk back to the other.

What does it all mean?

Understanding pupillary changes

Use this chart as a guide to pupillary changes.

Pupillary change	Possible causes
Unilateral, dilated (4 mm), fixed, and nonreactive 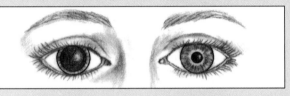	• Uncal herniation with oculomotor nerve damage • Brain stem compression • Increased intracranial pressure • Tentorial herniation • Head trauma with subdural or epidural hematoma • May be normal in some people
Bilateral, dilated (4 mm), fixed, and nonreactive 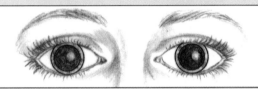	• Severe midbrain damage • Cardiopulmonary arrest (hypoxia) • Anticholinergic poisoning
Bilateral, midsize (2 mm), fixed, and nonreactive 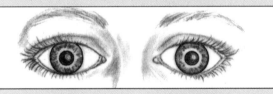	• Midbrain involvement caused by edema, hemorrhage, infarctions, lacerations, contusions
Bilateral, pinpoint (<1 mm), and usually nonreactive 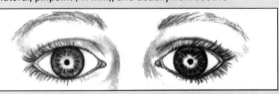	• Lesion of pons, usually after hemorrhage
Unilateral, small (1.5 mm), and nonreactive 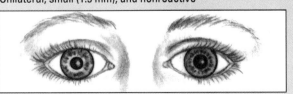	• Disruption of sympathetic nerve supply to the head caused by spinal cord lesion above the first thoracic vertebrae

Ptosis

Drooping of the eyelid, or ptosis, can result from a defect in the oculomotor nerve. To assess ptosis more accurately, have the patient sit upright.

Facial nerve impairment

If the patient responds inadequately to sensory stimulation of the skin or eye, the trigeminal nerve may be affected. Trigeminal neuralgia causes severe, lancinating pain over one or more of the facial dermatomes.

Auditory problems

Sensorineural hearing loss can result from lesions of the cochlear branch of the acoustic nerve or from lesions in any part of the nerves' pathway to the brain stem. A patient with this type of hearing loss may have trouble hearing high-pitched sounds or he may have a total loss of hearing in the affected ear.

Other problems

Vertigo is the illusion of movement and can result from a disturbance of the vestibular centers. If it's caused by a peripheral lesion, vertigo and nystagmus will occur 10 to 20 seconds after the patient changes position, and symptoms will gradually lessen with the repetition of the position change. If the vertigo is of central origin, there is no latent period, and the symptoms won't diminish with repetition.

Dysphagia, or difficulty swallowing, often occurs after a stroke but can also be the result of a mass lesion affecting cranial nerves IX and X.

Speech disorders

Aphasia is a speech disorder caused by injury to the cerebral cortex. Several types of aphasia exist, including:
• expressive or Broca's aphasia — impaired fluency and "word-finding" difficulty; impairment located in the frontal lobe, the anterior speech area
• receptive or Wernicke's aphasia — inability to understand written words or speech and the use of made-up words; impairment located in the posterior speech cortex, which involves the temporal and parietal lobes
• global aphasia — lack of both expressive and receptive language; impairment of both speech areas.

Constructional problems

Apraxia and agnosia are two types of constructional disorders.

What's the purpose of this?

Apraxia is the inability to perform purposeful movements and make proper use of objects. It's often associated with parietal lobe dysfunction and can appear in any of four types:

• ideomotor apraxia — loss of ability to understand the effect of a motor activity, ability to perform simple activities but without awareness of performing them, and an inability to perform actions on command

• ideational apraxia — awareness of actions that need to be done but inability to perform them

• constructional apraxia — inability to copy a design such as the face of a clock

• dressing apraxia — inability to understand the meaning of various articles of clothing or the sequence of actions required to get dressed.

What did you say this was?

Agnosia is the inability to identify common objects. It may indicate a lesion in the sensory cortex. Types of agnosia include:

• visual — inability to identify common objects unless they're touched

• auditory — inability to identify common sounds

• body image — inability to identify body parts by sight or touch, inability to localize a stimulus, denial of existence of half the body.

Abnormal muscle movements

Neurologic disorders can cause a wide range of abnormal muscle movements from facial tics to motor restlessness. Findings may or may not indicate serious neurologic disease.

Uncontrollable tics

These sudden, uncontrolled movements of the face, shoulders, and extremities are caused by abnormal neural stimuli. Tics are normal movements that appear repetitively and inappropriately. They include blinking, shoulder shrugging, and facial twitching.

Involuntary tremors

Like tics, tremors are involuntary, repetitive movements usually seen in the fingers, wrist, eyelids, tongue, and legs. They can occur when the affected body part is at rest or with voluntary movement. For example, the patient with Parkinson's disease has a characteristic "pill rolling" resting tremor, and the patient with cerebellar disease has an "intention tremor" as he reaches for an object.

Small muscle fasciculations

Fasciculations are fine twitchings in small muscle groups that are most commonly associated with lower motor neuron dysfunction.

Abnormal gaits

During your assessment, you may identify a gait abnormality. These may result from disorders of the cerebellum, posterior columns, corticospinal tract, basal ganglia, and lower motor neurons.

Hemiparetic gait

Characteristics of the hemiparetic gait vary according to the amount of upper motor neuron damage. In severe cases, the patient walks with the affected upper extremity abducted and the elbow, wrist, and fingers flexed. The upper body is somewhat stooped, and he tilts slightly to the opposite side. As he walks, he extends his legs and inverts his foot at the ankle. The leg swings in a circular motion.

Ataxic gait

Caused by cerebellar damage, an ataxic gait is wide-based and reeling; it's often called "drunken gait." If sensory loss occurs, the ataxia can result from the patient's not being able to feel where he's placing his foot.

In this gait pattern, the patient partially flexes his hips and lifts up his legs. He slaps his feet down with each step.

Steppage gait

In a steppage gait pattern, the patient purposely lifts up his legs and slaps them down on the floor. This gait is associated with lower motor neuron disease and is often accompanied by muscle weakness and atrophy.

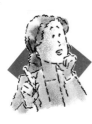

Quick quiz

1. Mental status screening questions are used at the beginning of a neurologic assessment in order to:

    A. elicit information about the cranial nerves.

    B. determine the patient's emotional status.

    C. assess level of orientation and the need for a more detailed examination.

Answer: C. Mental status screening questions are a quick way to discover disordered thought processes that might not be apparent when the patient answers questions requiring only a yes-or-no answer.

2. The most sensitive indicator of a change in a patient's neurologic status is his:

    A. gross motor movement.

    B. level of consciousness.

    C. speech patterns.

Answer: B. While gross motor movement and speech patterns may change with an alteration in neurologic status, LOC is the most sensitive and earliest indicator of this.

3. If a patient can't recognize the sound of a ringing phone, he probably has:

    A. agnosia.

    B. apraxia.

    C. aphasia.

Answer: A. Agnosia, or the inability to identify common objects, occurs in three forms: visual, auditory, or body image.

4. Normal findings in the assessment of gross motor function include:

    A. a smooth, coordinated gait.

    B. a positive Romberg's test.

    C. the ability to distinguish odors.

Answer: A. A smooth, coordinated gait is a normal gross motor finding; so is a negative Romberg's test.

5. One of the primitive reflexes is the:

    A. grasping reflex.

    B. patellar reflex.

    C. brachial reflex.

Answer: A. The grasping, snout, sucking, and glabella reflexes occur normally in infants, whose neurologic systems are immature, but they're abnormal in adults.

6. Equipment used to test sensation includes a:
    A. key and tongue blade.
    B. safety pin and cotton wisp.
    C. pencil and paper.

Answer: B. A safety pin and cotton wisp are used to assess pain and light touch.

Scoring

☆☆☆   If you answered all six items correctly, wow! Your cerebral cortex is working overtime and you qualify for a membership in the International Association of Class A Neurons!

☆☆   If you answered four or five items correctly, fantastic! Your gait is so steady, you finished first in the North American Neurologic Diencephalon!

☆   If you answered fewer than four items correctly, no problemo! You fine-tuned your reflexes and entered the National League for a Higher Level of Consciousness!

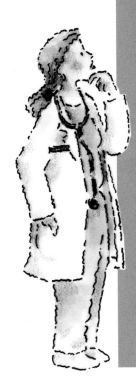

Glossary and index

Glossary

accommodation: a change in the shape of the lens that allows the eye to focus on a nearby object; accompanied by constriction of the pupils and convergence of the eyes

adnexa: appendages of the uterus, including ovaries, fallopian tubes, and supporting tissues

alert: term used to describe a patient who can follow commands, comprehends verbal and written language, is able to express ideas freely, and is oriented to time, place, and person

alopecia: hair loss

amplitude: strength of a pulse or other force that's recorded as bounding, normal, weak, or absent

anisocoria: unequal pupils

ankylosis: fixation of a joint due to fibrous or bony union; results from a disease process

anorexia: loss of appetite

anthropometric measurements: measurements of the human body performed as part of a comprehensive nutritional assessment; include midarm circumference, skin-fold thickness, and midarm muscle circumference

aphasia: language disorder, difficulty in expressing or comprehending speech

apraxia: inability to perform coordinated movements, even though there is no motor deficit

ascites: accumulation of fluid in the abdominal cavity

ataxia: uncoordinated actions of voluntary muscle use

auscultation: physical assessment technique in which the examiner listens (usually with a stethoscope) for sounds coming from the heart, lungs, abdomen, or other organs

bimanual palpation: method of palpation using two hands to locate body structures and assess their texture, size, consistency, mobility, and tenderness

borborygmus: loud, gurgling, splashing sounds normally heard over the large intestine and caused by gas passing through the intestine

bruit: abnormal sound heard over peripheral vessels that indicates turbulent blood flow

cardiac cycle: the period from the beginning of one heartbeat to the beginning of the next; includes two phases, systole and diastole.

cataract: opacity of the lens of the eye

cerumen: waxlike secretion in the external ear

closed questions: questions that elicit yes-or-no answers

coma: unconscious state in which the patient appears to be asleep and doesn't speak or respond to body or environmental stimuli

consensual light reflex: reflex constriction of the pupil of one eye when the other eye is illuminated

cremasteric reflex: superficial reflex in men; elicited by stroking the upper inner thigh, which causes brisk retraction of the testis on the side of the stimulus

crepitus: noise or vibration produced by rubbing together irregular cartilage surfaces or broken ends of a bone; also the sound heard when air in subcutaneous tissue is palpated

dimpling: puckering or depression of the skin of the breast possibly caused by underlying growth; also called retraction

diplopia: double vision

dorsal lithotomy position: position commonly used for female pelvic examinations in which the patient lies on her back with her hips and knees flexed and her thighs abducted and rotated externally

dysarthria: speech defect often related to a motor deficit of the tongue or speech muscles

Erb's point: auscultatory point on the precordium located at the third intercostal space to the left of the sternum

exophthalmos: abnormal protrusion of the eyeball

expressive aphasia: difficulty or inability to express words or thoughts

flaccidity: decreased muscle tone, which causes muscle to become weak or flabby

fluid wave: rippling seen across the abdomen when percussed; indicative of the presence of ascites

fremitus: palpable vibration that results from air passing through the bronchopulmonary system and transmitting vibrations to the chest wall

gynecomastia: enlargement of breast tissue in a male

heave: strong outward thrust palpated over the chest during systole; also called lift

hernia: abnormal protrusion of a structure through an opening, such as when a loop of bowel protrudes through a muscle wall

hirsutism: excessive hair growth that may be a sign of an endocrine disorder, heredity, or the effect of certain drugs

hordeolum: inflammation of the sebaceous gland of the eyelid; also called stye

hydrocele: accumulation of serous fluid in a saclike structure such as the testis

hyperopia: defect in vision that allows a person to see objects clearly at a distance but not at close range; also called farsightedness

hyperresonance: increased resonance produced by percussion

inspection: critical observation of the patient during physical assessment in which the examiner may use sight, hearing, or smell to make informed observations

intensity: degree of strength; for example, the loudness of a heart murmur recorded as soft, medium, or loud

introitus: entrance into the vagina

jaundice: yellowish discoloration of the skin caused by the accumulation of bilirubin

kwashiorkor: protein-deficiency malnutrition that occurs in young children and involves a loss of visceral protein

lethargy: slowed responses, sluggish speech, and slowed mental and motor processes in a person oriented to time, place, and person

lichenification: thickening of the skin related to eczema that occurs especially in the antecubital and popliteal fossae

mammogram: X-ray of the breast used to detect tumors and other abnormalities

marasmus: protein and calorie malnutrition that primarily affects children ages 6 to 18 months; results from a chronic lack of nutrients

meatus: opening or passageway in the body

menarche: first menstrual period

menopause: cessation of the menstrual period

murmur: abnormal sound heard on auscultation of the heart; caused by abnormal blood flow through a valve

mydriasis: dilation of the pupil due to paralysis of the oculomotor muscles or the effects of drugs

myopia: defect in vision that allows a person to see objects clearly at close range but not at a distance; also called nearsightedness

nipple inversion: inward turning or depression of the central portion of the nipple

nystagmus: involuntary, rhythmic movement of the eyes

objective data: information verifiable through direct observation, laboratory tests, screening procedures, or physical examination

occult blood: blood hidden in stool or urine that can be detected with a guaiac test

open-ended question: question that requires an answer in a sentence form rather than a yes-or-no response

palpation: physical assessment technique in which the examiner uses the sense of touch to feel pulsations and vibrations or to locate body structures and assess their texture, size, consistency, mobility, and tenderness

peau d'orange: orange-peel appearance of breast skin caused by edema; associated with breast cancer

percussion: physical assessment technique in which the examiner taps on the skin surface with his fingers to assess the size, border, and consistency of internal organs and to detect and evaluate fluid in a body cavity

peristalsis: sequence of muscle contractions that propels food through the GI tract

pitch: frequency of a sound, measured in the number of sound waves generated per second

point of maximal impulse (PMI): point at which the upward thrust of the heart against the chest wall is greatest, usually over the apex of the heart

precordium: area of the chest over the heart

protein-calorie malnutrition (PCM): spectrum of disorders resulting from either prolonged or chronic inadequate protein or calorie intake or from high metabolic requirements for protein and energy

pruritus: severe itching

ptosis: drooping of the eyelid

rebound tenderness: sharp, stabbing pain that occurs when the abdomen is pushed in deeply and then suddenly released; usually associated with peritoneal inflammation

receptive aphasia (fluent aphasia): inability to understand the spoken word

resonance: clear, hollow, low-pitched sound produced by percussion; typically heard over normal lungs

strabismus: lack of coordination of eye muscles

striae: stripes or lines of tissue differing in color and texture from the surrounding tissue

stupor: state in which a patient lies quietly with minimal spontaneous movement and is unresponsive except to vigorous and repeated stimuli

subjective data: information that the patient, his family, or his friends give to the health care provider about the patient's current health care status during the health history; reflects the personal perspective of patient, family, and friends

synovial joint: type of freely movable joint lined with a synovial membrane that secretes synovial fluid for lubrication

tail of Spence: extension of breast tissue that projects from the upper outer quadrant of the breast toward the axilla

telangiectasis: permanently dilated small blood vessels that form a weblike pattern; may be the result of scleroderma, lupus erythematosus, or cirrhosis or may be normal in healthy, older adults

thrill: palpable vibration felt over the heart or vessel that results from turbulent blood flow

tinnitus: ringing sound in one or both ears

tone: normal degree of vigor and tension; in muscle, the normal degree of tension

tympany: musical, drumlike sound heard normally when percussing over a hollow organ such as the stomach

vertigo: illusion of the movement of a patient's body or surroundings

vitiligo: areas of complete absence of melanin pigment leading to patchy areas of white or light skin

Index